Researching Health Needs

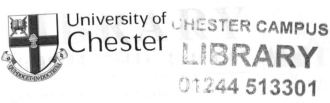

University of CHESTER CAMPUS
Chester LIBRARY
01244 513301

D1345020

Researching Health Needs

A Community-based Approach

Judy Payne

SAGE Publications

London · Thousand Oaks · New Delhi

© Judy Payne 1999

First published 1999

 SAGE Publications Ltd
6 Bonhill Street
London EC2A 4PU

SAGE Publications Inc
2455 Teller Road
Thousand Oaks, California 91320

SAGE Publications India Pvt Ltd
32, M-Block Market
Greater Kailash-I
New Delhi 110 048

British Library Cataloguing in Publication data

A catalogue record for this book is available from the
British Library

ISBN 0 7619 6083 X
ISBN 0 7619 6084 8 (pbk)

Library of Congress catalog card number 99–072823

Typeset by Type Study, Scarborough, North Yorkshire
Printed by The Cromwell Press Ltd, Trowbridge, Wiltshire

For Charlie

CONTENTS

LIST OF TABLES

LIST OF FIGURES

PREFACE

The idea of writing a user-friendly book about how to do health and social research has its origins in work I did for the Healthy Plymouth Alliance. The Alliance needed a short handbook on the techniques used in health needs assessment of local communities. It was designed as a practical guide that could be used both by professionals and directly by local community groups. While preparing the handbook, it became clear that there was a need for a more detailed and extensive text. Although this would still be user-friendly and practical in style, it could also be used by students on undergraduate and post-qualification courses in health, community work, social care and social science, and by practising professionals.

The result is this book, which sets out ways of doing social research into community-based health issues. In one sense, it is a book about *social* research, in which the examples and the development of the ideas are taken largely from community health. Viewed in this way, it should be helpful for anyone learning about social research: the methods described are equally used in sociology and social policy. In another sense, it is a book about *health*, and ways of thinking about it and investigating it. Based in a framework of local people and processes, it seeks to avoid a 'medical model' of health and illness, and to take account of the complexity of human life, agencies and policies.

It covers all the main methods that have been used to research health in local communities, beginning with the more straightforward and practical steps. I have tried to start with common sense issues, and to show how these are often a little more complicated than they seem. In the same way, doing research often entails specific procedures (and harder work!) than might appear to be the case at first sight. The aim throughout is to give enough information to enable research to be done, without going overboard on the technicalities.

Because the book tries to avoid being too technical, it also indicates the points in doing research when more specialist help should be obtained. Thirty years of doing research and teaching social research methods (much of it in a health setting) have shown me that we cannot all be equally expert in everything. Doing good health research, and doing it confidently, entails recognizing what we can do, and when we need to call on the skills of other professionals.

The result is a pragmatic book, dealing with the practicalities of how to do research, from first thoughts through to writing it up, getting the message out, and trying to influence health and social policies. What I have drawn together are methods from a range of perspectives. Some of these are conventionally called 'qualitative', while others are 'quantitative'. In practice, the boundary between them is less clear-cut than most texts imply. Underlying research is a way of thinking through questions systematically, and then choosing the appropriate techniques to carry it out.

It follows that the book has a core approach that is developed and worked through in each chapter. Each chapter starts with an overview, describes a number of methods, both in terms of practical steps and their advantages and disadvantages, and concludes with a practice exercise and a reminder of key concepts and terms. Examples of recent studies are included, so that the principles can be seen in concrete form. Details of case studies, a glossary and sources are included at the end of the book. Many of the chapters can be taken as free-standing, so that readers will be able to follow their own order or selection of methods through most of the book. It certainly has not been constructed to be read from cover to cover in one sitting, and some of the more detailed sections will repay re-reading.

Although I might have eventually got round to writing this book, it was my work for the Healthy Plymouth Alliance that led me to doing it now. The HPA Board members gave me every encouragement during the preparation of the original handbook. In particular, Maggie Grant, the Co-ordinator of HPA was always supportive and enthusiastic. During the writing, I have been fortunate that my partner, Geoff Payne, is also a Professor of Sociology and health researcher at the University of Plymouth, and my sister, Dr Jennifer Roberts, a Reader in the Department of Public Health and Policy at the London School of Hygiene and Tropical Medicine. They contributed a very welcome resource of personal and professional support. I would also like to acknowledge past and present colleagues and students in Newcastle, Aberdeen and Plymouth, in whose company I have developed my own understanding of the processes of social research. Finally, I am grateful to Karen Phillips and Kiren Shoman for their advice during the preparation of this book for Sage.

CHAPTER I

INTRODUCTION

Despite the many changes to the NHS in the 1990s, successive governments have drawn on two underlying principles in planning and resource allocation. First, allocation strategies and practice should be based on the best available information and evidence. Second, health authorities should consult and inform their local populations about needs and priorities. Thus, Mawhinney's statement that 'decisions must be based on sound evidence about health needs' (1993: 18) was echoed four years later by Jay when announcing the publication of the Department of Health's *Policy Research Programme*:

> it [is] vital that government policy [is] based on thorough investigation and proven evidence . . . Research and development plays a crucial role in providing information on a wide range of issues that will enable us to improve the quality of services on which the health and well-being of the whole population depends. (Department of Health, 1997c)

Similarly, the importance of local consultation put forward in *Local Voices* (NHS Management Executive, 1992) is repeated in the 1997 White Paper 'Health Authorities will need to: involve the public in developing the Health Improvement Programme' (Department of Health, 1997a: para 4.19). The Health Action Zones announced in this White Paper are partnerships of local statutory authorities, voluntary organizations and local people working together to develop 'innovative strategies' to improve health in their area.

The two underlying principles of evidence-based planning and practice, and local consultation and involvement are brought together most clearly in the requirement that health authorities undertake *health needs assessments* of their local populations. This was made a statutory duty in the 1990 NHS and Community Care Act, and reinforced in the 1997 White Paper. The first 'key task' of health authorities is '**assessing the health needs** of the local population, drawing on the knowledge of other organisations' (Department of Health, 1997a: para 4.3). However, although the National Health Service Management Executive (NHSME) recommended a possible approach to carrying out these assessments (NHS Management Executive, 1991), a wide variety of techniques and methods have been used. These range from the calculation of mortality and morbidity rates for different diseases (an *epidemiological* approach), through QALYs – quality-adjusted life year estimates (an *economics* approach), to social surveys, focus groups, forums and less formal discussions and observations in local communities (a *sociological* approach).

This book provides a description of the main methods used in *sociological approaches* to community needs assessments and community health profiling. All of the methods discussed here are 'tried and tested'. They have been employed by sociologists and others for many years – some for more than half a century. Often they have been used in combination – a *mixed-method* or *triangulation* approach – to get information about different aspects of a topic or to validate the results of other methods.

Selecting which methods to use is largely determined by the nature of the research question (what you want to find out) and the available resources. In addition, it will depend on the particular theoretical perspective and goals of the researcher. In finding out about the health needs of local populations, this will involve what definitions of 'community', 'health' and 'need' are used, and why the research is being undertaken.

This first chapter provides a framework for the detailed discussions of these methods in later chapters. As we shall see, these apparently familiar and straightforward words hide a complex set of conflicting meanings once we begin to unpack them. First, we will look at the different meanings of the terms 'community', 'health' and 'need'. This is followed by a discussion of the research process and the different research strategies – what 'doing research' involves. Again, we will discover that what at first sight seems common sense and easy, actually is a technical and sometimes challenging set of activities.

What do we mean by 'community', 'health' and 'needs'?

Health needs assessments of communities are descriptions of the 'health states' and 'needs' of the people belonging to those communities. Within the NHS, they are currently defined as

> The process by which a Health Authority *uses* information to judge the health of its population and then determine what services should be provided locally. (NHS Executive, 1998: 121; emphasis added)

This is an extremely exclusive definition in that it refers to 'use' rather than information collection. Further, it restricts the process to activities carried out within the NHS, and health authorities in particular. However, many community groups and local health alliances (for example, many *Healthy Cities* projects) have undertaken health assessments and health profiles of their communities. This information has first been collected using many of the methods discussed in the following chapters and then *used* as part of the assessment process. The definition offered by the National Health Service Executive (NHSE, the successor to the NHSME) also carries the implication that only health authorities can determine what services are provided, but we can all have our own views on this. Moreover, by avoiding any definitions of 'health' and 'needs', the NHSE carefully sidesteps what Foreman (1996) has termed 'complex and contestable' conceptual issues. In addition, it defines the appropriate population group as that covered by each local health authority. In contrast, many health needs assessments have covered different community groupings.

Community

In everyday usage, **community** is often used to refer to the population of a geographically defined location. In contrast to **locality** which refers to the geographical area, *community* emphasizes the social dimensions that result from living in a particular location, especially the shared values, aims and actions of a population group. However, the term is often used to refer not just to the resident population but also to those who take part in or have an impact on its social life: those who work there, for example, but live elsewhere.

Again, communities may be made up of groups of people who come together for a certain purpose: for example, a school, a work group or a hospital – *institution-based* communities. Further, *community* need not necessarily be restricted to a particular locality or site. Groups of people who share some common interest or characteristic may be regarded as *communities of interest*: for example, the Anglican community, the Black community, mother and baby groups, Manchester United supporters.

Although these concepts of *community* convey ideas of social cohesion, cooperation and solidarity, this is not always the case. It is likely that any one community will be composed of members of other communities. For example, a locality-based community will consist of people who belong to different work-based communities, ethnic communities, religious communities, political communities etc. Such *overlapping communities* are therefore likely to experience a range of disagreements and conflicts amongst their members.

An important aspect of the concept of *community* is that of a group of *people recognizing that they have something in common*. Unless they do, they can only be regarded as a 'potential' community: a group of people who are seen from the outside as a community but who do not themselves feel that they share a common identity or have a need to cooperate. Community development is the process by which this identity and cooperation is encouraged.

Any studies that focus on communities will have to take account of these various dimensions in determining the most appropriate approach(es) to be adopted.

Health

We use the word *health* in many ordinary conversations: about people – 'what a *healthy*-looking baby'; about ideas and things – 'that's a *healthy* attitude to take'; and about the environment – 'it's a very *healthy* place to live'. In all of these examples *health* is used to mean a positive characteristic or state: good as opposed to bad. On the other hand, in the medical context, *health* is defined negatively in terms of the absence of disease, impairment, disability or handicap. This approach is illustrated by the way in which the health of the population is assessed by comparing death rates and disease occurrences over time and between groups (*epidemiology*). For example, an examination of data used to monitor government targets and those included in public health reports shows that many of the main indicators of *health* are *death rates* and *illness rates*.

This very narrow medical definition of health is gradually being replaced by a more positive and broad concept: *health as well being*. As early as 1948, the World Health Organization (WHO) included in its constitution the statement that 'Health is a state of complete physical, social and mental well being'. Here, health is seen not just as the absence of disease but is also associated with the *quality of life*. Thus the 1997 White Paper recognized this distinction in setting out a new vision of 'an NHS that does not just treat people when they are ill but works with others to improve health and health inequalities' (Department of Health, 1997a: para 1.1). This wider (*holistic*) definition includes the social, economic and environmental circumstances that affect people's ability to experience a healthy life. The influence of such factors as unemployment, occupation and residence on death and illness rates has been acknowledged since Victorian times within the public health movement, and the reduction/eradication of such inequalities was the guiding principle behind the introduction of the Welfare State in the 1940s. However, research carried out since the late 1970s shows that these inequalities still exist and are, if anything, increasing (see, for instance, Department of Health, 1998b).

The present Labour government has placed the reduction of these inequalities at the centre of its health policy. The 1998 Public Health Green Paper identified the many 'complex causes' of these inequalities some are *fixed* – ageing, for instance, or genetic factors [Others can be changed.] These include a range of factors to do with how we all live our lives – diet, physical activity, sexual behaviour, smoking, alcohol, and drugs [*lifestyle*]. *Social and economic* issues play a part too – poverty, unemployment and social exclusion. So too does our *environment* – air and water quality, and housing. And so does access to *good services*, like education, transport, social services and the NHS itself. (Department of Health, 1998a: 5; emphasis added)

There is a recognition here that health is not just a *medical* matter. Because of these differing views of what constitutes 'health', it is important to construct a working definition that states clearly what factors you mean to include before undertaking an investigation of health needs.

Needs

There is even less agreement about the definition of *need* than there is about *community* or *health*. Much of the literature on health need draws on a definition put forward more than twenty-five years ago that distinguished four types of need: *normative* (as defined by professionals/experts); *felt* (wants, wishes, desires); *expressed* (felt need turned into action or vocalized: for example, asking for pain relief, striking for more pay); and *comparative need* (inequalities) (Bradshaw, 1972).

These distinctions, although of value for clarification purposes, are of limited use when investigating the health needs of communities. Clearly, people's perceived health needs (felt needs) are influenced both by 'expert' definitions and by comparisons with the health states of other individuals and groups. Thus *need* may be defined in terms of comparative standards or inequalities. This is highlighted by the stress on inequalities in the Public Health Green Paper (Department of Health, 1998a).

An alternative approach is offered by Doyal and Gough in their book *A Theory of Human Need* (1991). The authors have developed a theory of universal human needs based on the basic requirements of physical health and personal independence (*autonomy*). These are achieved by satisfying what they term *intermediate needs*:

- adequate nutritional food and clean water
- adequate protective housing
- a non-hazardous work environment
- a non-hazardous physical environment
- appropriate health care
- security in childhood

- significant primary relationships (with family, friends, neighbours)
- physical security
- economic security
- appropriate education
- safe birth control and child-bearing.

The more detailed definitions of these intermediate needs are then determined at the national/local level. The main problem with the use of this theory in a needs assessment exercise is that of defining what is meant by 'adequate', 'appropriate', 'non-hazardous', 'significant' and 'safe'. These terms would have to be further clarified before any research based on this theory was undertaken. An example of the use of this theory of need can be found in a study of local needs carried out in Leeds in the early 1990s (Percy-Smith and Sanderson, 1992).

A further aspect of need concerns that of *satisfying* or meeting needs. This naturally concerns decisions about resource allocation and the setting of priorities that are basically political and ethical in nature (for example, should deprived areas have more money allocated to them than other areas?; should the treatment of certain illnesses have a higher priority than others?). Thus *need* has been defined for community care assessment purposes as 'the ability of an individual or collection of individuals *to benefit from care*' (Department of Health, 1993: 6; emphasis added). This contrasts with the statement in the 1997 White Paper where

> access to [the NHS] will be **based on need** and need alone – not on your ability to pay, or on who your GP happens to be or where you live. (Department of Health, 1997a: para 1.5)

Here *need* is not overtly defined. Later in the same chapter, there is the suggestion that it refers to felt or expressed need: 'responsive to the needs and preferences of the people who use [the services of the NHS]' (para 1.19). However, the same document also makes reference to decisions being 'best made by those who treat patients [but] set [in] a framework . . . to ensure consistency and fairness' (para 1.22).

Doing research

Doing research about a community or social group is, in many ways, an extension of what we do in our everyday lives. If we want to find out about something, we ask our friends what they think, we watch television or read newspapers and magazine articles. We then evaluate all of this information, selecting the most important and useful to us, in order to reach conclusions as a basis for some further action. The main difference between these everyday processes and the methods and techniques of social research is that the research process is far more structured and formalized.

Although social research may look easy, it is not. Social scientists have usually undergone extensive training in research skills before embarking on any major project themselves. The methods used to observe, ask questions, examine existing information and analyse the resulting data in social research have been rigorously developed and tested to form a systematic body of knowledge and techniques (sometimes called 'methodologies'). Further, the findings of the research are expected to be presented in a coherent and structured manner as a formal report that can be scrutinized by others.

This scrutiny often includes checking that the findings and the methods used to produce them are *valid* and *reliable*. Here, *validity* refers to accuracy and *reliability* refers to consistency. A related concept is that of *objectivity* or bias. 'Being objective' means approaching the research in an open-minded manner where one's own beliefs, values and prejudices affect neither the collection nor the interpretation of information. Complete objectivity is impossible to achieve, particularly in policy-related research. Instead, one attempts to produce credible and trustworthy evidence by being honest about one's biases and feelings (*reflexivity*), by examining the context, motivation and conduct of the research (*radical qualification*), and by allowing others to scrutinize the research (*peer review*). These issues are discussed in Chapter 3.

It will already be clear from the previous pages that researchers are operating in a context of competing political and intellectual ideas. A variety of positions can be taken as starting points, and these naturally influence what you do and what you think of as 'doing research'. These *theoretical orientations* are part and parcel of every researcher's approach. Even this book necessarily adopts a position, stressing practical ways of doing systematic research with a view to influencing policy, and treating qualitative and quantitative research techniques as equally valuable.

Some social scientists (and those less well qualified to comment) would reject the validity of this position. On the one hand, some might say that quantitative methods are no good, because we cannot count or measure human feelings. On the other hand, some writers dismiss anything but scientific experiments as 'soft' unreliable ways of collecting information, open to bias by the researcher. A third group might claim that social research never changes policy: the rich (and healthy) get richer, the poor (and unhealthy) get poorer. This book regards such extreme positions as being far too narrow, and advocates careful, rigorous ways of studying the social world around us.

Unlike when we are dealing with 'everyday finding out', and whether we are adopting one of the extreme positions rejected here or the present pragmatic approach to social research, we need to confront the issue of *ethics* or *ethical research*. The professional organizations to which academic, government and market researchers belong have developed codes of conduct that govern research involving the public. Central to these codes is the principle of *informed consent*. This means that full information about the nature of the research should be given to people who are asked to take part, and their right to refuse and their privacy must be respected (and for those under 18, this means the permission of a parent or guardian as well). Their *anonymity* and the *confidentiality* of the information they provide must also be ensured. This is achieved by separating the information that people give (on questionnaires, in interviews etc.) from their identity by using code numbers rather than names. However, some research methods prevent complete anonymity (for example, focus groups, video interviews), and in such cases permission must be obtained.

A final issue concerns the reasons for doing research: why are you doing your project? Usually this is to learn more about something either for its own sake (*research for knowledge*) or in order to do something (*research for action*). Investigations of health needs are likely to be for action of some kind. This could be to produce information – commissioned or in-house – that others can act upon: for instance, resource allocation, policy review or policy/practice evaluation. Alternatively, it could be that you want to highlight the concerns and needs of a particular group or area: *advocacy* or to bring about change. A further reason could be that your project is part of a community development strategy in which community participation and empowerment are the goals. Whatever your reasons, they should be clarified at the start of your research.

Stages of a research project

Research is perhaps best seen as a series of interlocking stages. First, the initial ideas have to be translated into a formal strategy or *research design* that is appropriate, manageable and practicable. This *planning stage* involves the clarification of the aims and objectives of the research through discussion, literature review and reflexivity. These are then translated into a central question or series of questions that can be investigated empirically within a specific theoretical and resource framework. Information is then *collected* using one or more methods. This information is then *analysed* using techniques that are appropriate to the type of information that has been collected. The analysis stage will generate *findings* that are then *presented* to a wider audience. The collection and analysis stages are often iterative in that questions that arise from the preliminary stages of analysis generate further information collection.

How to use this book

This book follows the research model described above, using examples from existing research to illustrate specific techniques and issues. Chapter 2 discusses the concerns and tasks that need to be addressed when planning research. This is followed by an introduction to the main methods of collecting information, and considers issues concerned with measurement, validity and reliability. Chapter 4 discusses the use of existing information and describes the main sources for this, including using the Internet.

Chapters 5–8 cover techniques for collecting new information. First, methods of selecting from whom to collect information are reviewed in Chapter 5. This is followed by discussions of the ways that questions are asked (Chapter 6) and observations made (Chapter 7). Chapter 8 reviews some of the recent tools and packages devised to investigate health needs. This chapter also introduces longitudinal studies and evaluative research.

The final three chapters are concerned with the analysis and presentation stages. Quantitative analysis is discussed in Chapter 9, and includes worked examples of the most common statistical techniques, while Chapter 10 describes methods used to analyse qualitative information. Finally, Chapter 11 gives an account of the ways that research findings are presented using formal reports, meetings and exhibitions. A brief description of some of the main studies used to illustrate the various techniques is given at the end, along with a Glossary of technical terms.

The book is not meant to be read from cover to cover. It is a textbook to help you 'do it yourself'. If you are reading it as part of a taught course, read the chapters relating to particular topics as they come up. If you are reading the book to help you do an independent project, read one or two chapters, take a break and then come back to it again. Get a sense of what is covered and discuss it with your group, colleagues, friends or family. At the end of each chapter is a summary which shows 'key words' in italics and you should make sure that you become familiar with them. Exercises are also given at the end of each chapter except the first two. They are designed to help you understand the various issues and techniques discussed before you do your own project 'for real'.

CHAPTER 2

PLANNING YOUR PROJECT

This chapter discusses how you might go about planning your project. The planning stage is crucial for the success of the project, and the amount of time needed to plan is often underestimated. Psychologically, collecting information is more rewarding than planning how it will be done. However, careful planning and preliminary data gathering (using existing sources of information) can save a lot of time later on. Further, if you intend to apply for funding, you will need to undertake a considerable amount of preparatory work before making any grant applications. In this chapter it is assumed that your research is being undertaken as a group initiative. However, even if you plan to do a small scale project on your own, you will still need to carry out many of the various tasks described here.

The first task in carrying out a health needs assessment project is to establish a framework for undertaking it. Obviously, this framework will be determined by the motivation for doing the assessment, the nature of your organization or group and the type and size of the community – whether it is locality- or interest-based. However, given these variations, it is possible to lay out some general guidelines about the activities that should be carried out at the outset.

One of the first steps when undertaking any research project is to set up a *steering group* to be responsible for the initial planning and refining of the project. Initially, the steering group's main task is to establish clear *aims and objectives*, and to set priorities within time, cost and other resource constraints. Once these have been clarified it will be necessary to consider *the methods* that you might use to collect the required information. These processes are covered in the first part of the chapter.

This is followed by a discussion of the methods of *involving the wider community* in your study. This includes the problems that might be faced, such as raising expectations and maintaining interest. Closely related to these issues is that of information dissemination. For instance, you will need to decide who you are going to inform, what action – if any – you will take, and which are the best methods of providing *feedback* to any sponsors and to the community itself.

In the final part of the chapter we examine the methods and problems involved in using external specialists. It is unlikely that you will need to consider their use in the first projects that you undertake. However, in your professional practice, you may be involved in large or complicated projects that are beyond the capabilities of a small team. In such instances it is usual to involve social research consultants. Before using consultants, you will need to specify their role and consider the tasks that they might undertake. This is easier once you have mastered what is involved in the research process.

Establishing a steering group

A steering group is responsible for the initial planning and management of the project. Its members should all have a commitment to the research, but should not necessarily have the same views. In fact, the success of the project will often depend on members being representative of the whole range of interests and opinions within a community. Ideally, therefore, the group should consist of people who are able to work together and respect each others' knowledge and differing opinions without necessarily agreeing on everything. The steering group should not be much larger than about eight members and could be smaller. The tasks that it will need to undertake are, for the most part, not suited to large group meetings. These larger groups usually require highly formal structures and inhibit free and frank discussions. If more people than this are keen to be involved, it is probably best to create sub-groups, responsible for particular aspects of the project.

There are a variety of ways of setting up a steering group. It could be that members are selected from your institution or organization. If your project is part of an educational course, your tutors will certainly need to be involved, and all necessary ethical procedures carried out. In addition, and particularly if the community is locality-based, you may want to involve the wider community or representatives from various interest groups and organizations. These might include public agencies (local authority, health authority, police, for example), political representatives and members of local voluntary organizations and community groups. If you decide to involve these wider groupings, you will need to decide how to approach the various organizations. This could be informally, through a series of meetings with individual interest groups, with a representative of a group, or by holding a single public meeting.

When arranging a public meeting it is important to decide on methods of publicizing the event: notices in local papers, shops, community centres etc. and leafleting are all appropriate. A suitable time should be fixed and a meeting place should be booked that is easily accessible. The date, time and venue should be shown clearly on any notices, in addition to a brief summary of the purpose of the meeting. If you decide to hold a representative meeting, letters and/or phone calls are more appropriate than public notices. But here again you must state clearly the purpose, venue and time of the meeting, and always allow sufficient notice. Before this initial meeting you will need to decide who will introduce the project, and to have a list of topics ready for discussion. Do not get despondent if only a small number of people attend. Many people do not attend meetings because of physical disabilities, lack of transport, or employment or child care commitments. Usually the aim of this first meeting is to ascertain support for the project, to determine general concerns and find suitable members of your steering group.

Once membership has been decided, the first task of the steering group should be to decide how it will operate: will there be a formal structure with a chairperson, secretary and agenda or will it be less structured; how often should it meet; where will it meet; and who will be responsible for any room bookings and notification of meetings. Often initiatives fail because these decisions are not taken at the outset. Once these organizational arrangements are made, the main priority of the group is to refine the general ideas into a manageable programme. This will entail setting aims, objectives and priorities; ascertaining and planning resources (time, skills, finance, personnel); allocating responsibilities; deciding on the methods to use; developing possible action strategies; and considering whether you need to use consultants.

Setting aims, objectives and priorities

At an early stage you will need to decide what exactly you want to do and why. It is not enough to say that you want to do a health needs assessment of a community in order to find out about people's health needs. First, you must *define the boundaries* of the community, whether it is locality-based or interest-based. If it is locality-based, you will need a large scale map of the area on which to draw the limits of your community. This exercise is of interest in itself in comparing people's mental maps of their community. If the community is interest-based, you will need to decide who exactly you are going to include: just members of your group or all of those who might be eligible. A further issue, which will be discussed in Chapter 5, is that of defining your population 'units' – individual people, households or particular age groups, for instance.

Setting the aims and objectives of the project is, arguably, the most important stage of the planning process. The aims of the project are the answers to the 'Why are we doing this project?' question. In setting aims, the steering group must reach a clear consensus on what the main purposes of the exercise are. For example, is it to influence resource allocation, to highlight a target group or to raise the consciousness of local people to health issues. Objectives are the more specific methods of achieving the aims.

The following extract from the Glasgow Healthy City Project starts with the aims, and then goes on to the objectives.

> The aim of the project is to make Glasgow a healthier city through joint work by the community, statutory and voluntary agencies. The objectives for the next five years are:
>
> - The development and implementation of a collaborative Health Plan for the City.
> - Support models of work at both local and policy level that illustrate the principles of 'Health for All'.
> - Develop work on food and poverty issues across the city with particular focus on access and supply.
> - Support the work of the Working Groups.
> - Develop new partnerships for health in the city. (Laughlin and Black, 1995: 118)

Although objectives are more specific than aims, they are not all equally specific. For instance, in the Glasgow example, the first objective will result in the publication of a document stating 'the plan' once it has been developed. On the other hand, objectives involving 'support' might result in something concrete like a document or finance, but equally could mean moral support and encouragement. Sometimes it is necessary to specify the objectives in such a way that their successful achievement can be measured and evaluated.

Once the aims and objectives of the project have been decided, they might then have to be prioritized. Setting priorities means deciding on what issues are most important in relation to the resources available to the project. These are not necessarily all related to financial matters, although having sufficient funds can overcome other shortfalls. Also, do not try to do too much. The Glasgow Healthy City example was carried out with the financial and personal support of the health and local authorities. For a smaller community project with much more limited resources, you should focus on only one or two main issues.

Selecting appropriate methods

Once the aims and objectives have been defined, it will be possible to determine the type and range of information that you will need and the most appropriate methods of collecting it. At this stage it is worth finding out what information already exists in the form of official reports and studies. Examining existing sources is a very useful way of clarifying what information you need to collect and the methods you might use. They may also help in identifying problems and pitfalls. The use of existing information is discussed in Chapter 4.

If the information that you need is not all available, it will be necessary to collect it directly. The methods used to collect new information can be broadly divided into *quantitative* and *qualitative*. Quantitative techniques are those used to obtain information that can be counted in some way (for example, how many people use the local health centre) and usually involve undertaking surveys. Qualitative techniques are used to get detailed information about people's feelings, experiences etc. (for example, an account of her daily life by an elderly woman). A mixed-method approach is often adopted in which both qualitative and quantitative techniques are used. The methods that you choose to use will determine what types of analyses are required. They are discussed in more detail in later chapters.

A further factor to be considered is the general nature of your project. Is it a one-off study that will be used for a particular purpose or is it part of a wider programme of action? You might want to evaluate the impact of certain changes or initiatives. In this case you will need to consider whether to study what the situation was like before the changes and then afterwards – a 'before/after' study, or whether to monitor the process over a longer period of time – a 'longitudinal' study. These issues are all important in the choice of techniques that you use and the resources that you will need. Evaluations and longitudinal studies are discussed in Chapter 8.

One example of these early stages in the setting up of a project is a community survey that was undertaken as part of a wider community participation project in the Winnall Manor Estate, Winchester. The project was funded by North and Mid Hampshire Health Commission and Winchester City Council. After funding was agreed, the Winchester *Health for All* coordinator invited a small group of representatives from voluntary and statutory agencies to form a steering group to plan the initial stages of the project. This involved identifying an appropriate locality and making contact with key individuals within it. Winnall Manor was selected because of its lack of community facilities and support structures. The key contact was a project worker from the Winchester Families Project who made contacts with residents and local mother and children groups.

A public meeting was arranged by residents and volunteers. This was attended by representatives of local organizations and agencies and local residents. As well as highlighting the lack of community facilities, those attending the meeting felt that there was a lack of information about community resources and needs. By the third meeting it was decided that a survey of community needs should be undertaken.

A survey planning group, consisting of local residents and organizational representatives with appropriate experience and knowledge, was set up. The following account describes the initial planning phase of this survey.

Background
The Winnall Community Survey Group was formed following the public meeting in May 1993. For the purposes of planning, implementation and evaluation of the survey, the group met on nine separate occasions between May and October 1993. A total of six residents were represented on the group working in collaboration with the Children's Society project worker, Health for All coordinator, and Families Support worker. Two student volunteers also attended the meetings on several occasions. Although individual attendance fluctuated slightly, there was always between two and four residents attending each meeting. The majority of meetings were held in the Community Centre. Administrative support for the meetings and the survey was provided by the Children's Society, the Health for All Coordinator and Mount Pleasant Media Workshop and Multi Media (Business Support).

Aim
The aim of the survey was to focus on the existing concerns highlighted in the three public meetings held between January and May 1993 and to provide a clearer picture of existing resources and priority concerns in Winnall. Concerns included: the environment, transport, facilities and leisure, health, safety and information. In addition it was hoped that the survey would also identify opportunities for promoting existing support networks and providing ideas for new activities on the Winnall estate. (Winnall Neighbourhood Forum, 1993: 13)

Checklists and timetables

Once you have decided on the research techniques, you should be able to draw up a list of your resource needs and an outline task timetable. Existing guides give examples of these (see Burton, 1993; Compass, 1996; Hawtin et al., 1994). However, it is important that such examples are not used rigidly. Any list you construct must relate to the needs and format of your project. A resource checklist should include the human, financial and equipment resources and requirements of your project. Resources needed are likely to include accommodation, furniture, personnel and time, skills, equipment (computer/word processor, photocopier, telephone, video, camera, tape recorder etc.) and transport. These should all be estimated at the planning stage so that full costings can be made and possible funding sources identified. A general outline of a checklist is given in Figure 2.1.

A task timetable or schedule is usually in the form of a list or grid,

Resources	Essential	Available	To get	Costs
People General Skills/experts Key contacts				
Accommodation Office Meetings Presentations Crèche				
Transport Fieldwork Respondents				
Equipment *Machines* Telephone Computer/printer Typewriter/calculator Photocopier Camera Video Tape recorder *Consumables* Stationery Stamps/postage Film Video cassettes Audio cassettes Computer software Maps Existing reports, statistics etc.				
Miscellaneous Printing Refreshments Expenses Electricity/telephone etc. Contingency/petty cash				

NB: This should be used as a guide only. Your list will be determined by the needs of your particular project.

Figure 2.1 *Resource and budget checklist*

but need not necessarily take this form. As an alternative you could use a *flow chart* (a chart that shows the relationships between tasks using arrows to indicate what comes next) or a 'year planner' chart with stick-on coloured shapes. On the other hand, you might find that you need an overall plan in one of these two formats and more detailed check-lists for individual or groups of tasks. In designing a timetable you first need to draw up a list of the tasks that have to be carried out, who will be responsible for them and an estimate of the time they will take. You will then have to work out the order in which they should be done. A general outline is given in Figure 2.2. This could be used as a frame-work, with more detailed tasks substituted as determined by your particular project.

For example, if you are intending to do a survey, you will need to

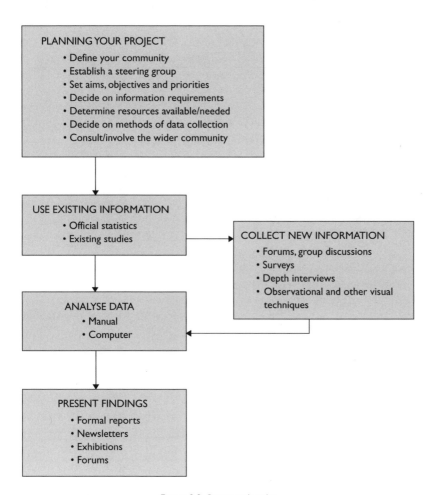

Figure 2.2 *Project task order*

Table 2.1. Example of the construction of a task timetable

Stage 1: Outline

Task	Responsibility	Time estimate
Sample	NP	2 weeks
Questionnaire design	CM/LJ and Group	10 weeks
Interviewing	TL	10 weeks
Processing	CM/LJ/NP	2 weeks
Analysis	CM/LJ and Group	4 weeks
Report	CM/LJ and Group	8 weeks

Stage 2: Individual task timetable for the first three tasks listed in Stage 1

Sampling	Interviewing	Questionnaire
Obtain population list – 1 day	Select interviewers – 2 weeks	Topic list – 2 weeks
Sample size – 1 day	Training – 2 weeks	Draft questionnaire – 3 weeks
Draw sample – 1 week	Brief for pilot – 1 day	Draft introductions/explanations – 1 week
Allocate interview lists – 3 days	Pilot draft questionnaire – 1 week	Print draft questionnaire – 3 days
	Pilot feedback – 1 day	Brief for pilot – 1 day
	Allocate interview lists – 3 days	Pilot draft questionnaire – 1 week
	Brief for survey – 1 day	Pilot feedback – 1 day
	Survey – 4 weeks	Revise questionnaire – 1 week
		Print questionnaire – 3 days
		Brief for survey – 1 day

Stage 3: Interlocking task timetable

Sampling	Interviewing	Questionnaire
		Topic list – 2 weeks
		Design questions, their order and coding frame – 3 weeks
		Draft introductions/explanations – 1 week
		Print first draft – 3 days
	Select interviewers – 2 weeks	
		Brief for piloting – 1 day
		Pilot draft 1 week
	Training – 2 weeks	Pilot feedback – 1 day
		Revise questionnaire – 1 week
		Print questionnaire – 3 days
	Brief for piloting – 1 day	
	Pilot draft – 1 week	
	Pilot feedback – 1 day	
Obtain full list of people – 1 day		
Decide on sample size – 1 day	Allocate list of names/addresses to interviewers – 3 days	
Draw sample – 1 week	Brief for final survey – 1 day	Brief for final survey – 1 day
Allocate list of names/addresses to interviewers – 3 days	Survey – 4 weeks	

select a sample, design a questionnaire, pilot it and print it, collect the information (by postal questionnaire or interviews), process and analyse the data, and write a report. If you decide to use interviewers, they will need to be selected, trained, briefed and de-briefed. Each task has then to be compared with the others so that the most appropriate timetable order is planned. The schedules shown in Table 2.1 illustrate the process.

In the Stage 1 part of the table, six tasks are identified in the left-hand column. For each, we can read across to see who will take responsibility for doing it, and how long it will take to complete. As the information given in Table 2.1 is not from an actual study, the initials in Stage 1 refer to imaginary people and you can substitute the initials of the people responsible for the tasks in your project. Obviously, if you are carrying out the project alone, you will not need this initials column. The Stage 2 part of the table illustrates three of the six tasks. Reading each column separately, we see the breakdown into sub-tasks and the time needed. Finally, in Stage 3, the order in which tasks have to be tackled begins to emerge as we read down and across each row in turn. The shaded areas in Stage 2 and 3 are the same, but the order, once they are interconnected, is different.

The times are not meant to be exact, but are just to show the broad timescales that these tasks might take. In Stage 2, the sub-tasks for sampling, interviewing and questionnaire design are listed separately, and those that are common to more than one of the main tasks are shaded. These, of course, are only carried out once. This table can then be used to map the timetable on to a calendar so that the common tasks interlock and are completed at the appropriate time.

Using the Stage 3 table in Table 2.1, we find, in this case, that the process would take approximately 14 weeks from starting to devise a topic list to completing the survey interviewing. Interview selection should begin by the middle of week 3 and the sampling process should start no later than the beginning of week 9. Of course, you may not be as tightly time-constrained in your research as in this example, and the actual times will be determined by your particular project. However, the example in Table 2.1 does illustrate how important it is to understand the relationships between tasks and how they interlock.

In drawing up timetables, you should always allow for your other commitments and those of others involved so that there are no hold-ups caused by employment, family, holidays and other activities. It is also important to monitor how the separate tasks are proceeding in case there are any hold-ups that impact on other tasks. And it is a good idea to include a week or two of 'slippage time' to allow for this. For instance, problems recruiting interviewers may delay the pilot stage and final survey timetable. The example here uses only three of the possible research tasks that you may carry out. In planning your project you will need to do this exercise for each of the tasks that you intend to undertake.

Involving the wider community

Whatever research strategy you adopt, it is now usual to involve the wider community in some way in your research. This is, of course, the essence of a participatory research strategy in which the researcher assists the community in the identification of its *own* needs. However, even here, not all members of a community will share your enthusiasm and commitment, although you are likely to find a good deal of support. For example, the Winnall project, discussed above, found that nearly 82 per cent of respondents to their survey did not want to be actively involved, although the majority were supportive.

Involving the wider community is thus likely to be more concerned with keeping people informed of what is happening and maintaining their support rather than encouraging their active participation – and too many volunteers could make the project unmanageable. Here, the contribution of the wider community is that of telling you what they think via public meetings, group discussions, surveys, etc. Consultation, as part of the research process and as feedback, is thus an important method of ensuring community interest and support. In this process you should not raise people's expectations about outcomes. It is essential to be honest about the project's aims and objectives, and any possible actions that may follow. Further, by approaching people as *local experts* rather than *objects of research*, you are more likely to obtain an accurate picture of the health needs of the community.

You will also need to decide when and how to inform the wider community and outside agencies (including funding bodies) about your findings. It might be more appropriate to provide a series of reports or feedbacks throughout the project rather than at the end, or you may want to do both. The decision will depend on such things as the length of time that it will take to carry out the project, the need to maintain interest and the need to keep a high profile. In addition to the timing of feedback, you should also consider the ways you will do it. Formal reports, meetings, news sheets, exhibitions and informal networking are among the various forms that feedback might take, and different methods can be used to inform different groups. These are discussed in Chapter 11.

Using experts/professionals

Undertaking a health needs project will require skills in such techniques as focus group facilitation, questionnaire design, interviewing and data manipulation and analysis. These, and many other necessary skills, are described in the following chapters. However, because they are predominantly practical skills, you will only become proficient by practising them. Furthermore, even when you have mastered the techniques involved, your professional practice may entail undertaking a research project that is far too demanding for you to undertake on your own. In this case, you will need help from others: colleagues, volunteers or social research practitioners. If you are attending a course, you will obviously seek help from your tutors.

Decisions about if and when to use experts to carry out your research are often based on resource factors. If funding is limited, there is usually no alternative but to undertake the research yourself with the help of colleagues and volunteers. You might be lucky enough to know people with some or all of the necessary skills who are willing to help out or give advice. Alternatively, you may decide that an important aspect of the project is to develop research skills within your organization and in the community itself. On the other hand, it is likely that the project will take much less time to complete, and will be more likely to be successful, if experts are involved in some or all of the processes. It might be that you decide that you have, or can acquire, some of the skills and will bring in a researcher to advise on or carry out other parts of the project. For example, you might ask a researcher to undertake discussion groups, while you will be responsible for questionnaire design and interviewing. Further, if you plan to use the results of your research to present a case to the local health authority or other public agencies, the research and the results need to be undertaken and presented in the most professional way possible.

Identifying people who have the necessary 'expert' knowledge and skills can also be a problem. Because you are concerned with *health* needs you may think that a medically qualified person might have the appropriate skills. However, a medical doctor is not usually trained in *social* research (unless he/she is a public health specialist). On the other hand, most health visitors have had some social research training. Lecturers at your local university or college who are specialists in sociology, social policy, community or social work will have studied courses in social research methods in their training. In addition, anyone who has graduated in these subjects might also be able to help. Even here, it is important to realize that not all will have the same depth of knowledge, understanding or aptitude. For example, two community development workers known to the author both admitted that they found their social research courses 'a struggle'. If you are unsure, it is probably best to contact an appropriate department at the nearest university or college and ask to be put in touch with a social research specialist. Also, organizations such as Community Health Councils and local health alliances might be able to give advice.

If you do decide to use a researcher for all or part of the project, you must establish clear guidelines about their part in the research and the nature of the contractual relationship. In these cases, it is usual to draw up a job specification (if you are employing them) or a tender document (if you intend to commission an independent researcher). This should state clearly what tasks you expect them to do; to whom they are responsible; the ownership (or copyright) of the results; any possible penalty clauses; and the financial arrangements. A guide to the market research rates for individual tasks is given in Table 2.2. Here you will see the high cost of such research expertise. However, consultancy rates at your local college or university are likely to be much lower than this.

Chapter summary

The planning stage is crucial for the success of your project. In this chapter we have discussed the issues involved in setting up a *steering group* and the *preliminary tasks* that need to be undertaken. Your steering group should have no more than eight members, but this is likely to be much smaller if your project is part of an academic course. One of the first tasks of this steering group is to clarify the nature of the project by setting *aims* and *objectives*. Aims are the overall goals of the project,

Table 2.2. *Market research costs*

Task	Cost
Consultants – discussion with clients, questionnaire design, analysis and report	£350–£500 per day
Focus Group organization	£700–£2,000 per group
Technical/administration – interview training, sampling, processing etc.	£250 per day
Interview survey – interview and data processed to machine readable format	£35–£50 per interview
Interviewer briefings	£1,500 per group of 6 interviewers

July 1996 costings.

The Market Research Society does not have standard rates. Each company decides their own charges. The above rates are based on quotations given by a number of companies.

while objectives are the more specific ways of achieving them. Once these have been decided, you will have to determine *what information* you will need and *what methods* you will use to collect it.

During this stage you will also have to review the *resources* that you will require to undertake the project, set *priorities* within your resource limits, and consider applying for *funding*. You should also think about how you might *involve the local community* and whether or not to *use a consultant*. Once these decisions are made, you will be in a position to *allocate tasks* and draw up a project *timetable*. The fieldwork stage, when you collect your information, can then begin.

CHAPTER 3

COLLECTING INFORMATION

Empirical social research, as discussed in Chapter 1, is concerned with using observable facts about the social world to explain, describe or understand it more clearly. The way we do this involves the selection, collection and analysis of information or evidence. However, unlike much of the information we use in our everyday lives, these processes are carried out *systematically*. The techniques and processes that are used have been developed to ensure that, as far as possible, our findings are justifiable.

This chapter provides an introduction to the principal methods that are used to produce empirical evidence – the selection and collection of information. First, it examines how this information (*data*) is defined and measured, and how we decide from where and from whom the information should be collected. Our choice will determine how far we can generalize from our findings to the wider social world. It then goes on to look at the range of techniques used to collect information, and their *applicability* to various research settings. When selecting what method to use to obtain information, we need to ensure that it is not only appropriate for our purposes but that it is also *valid* and *reliable*. These attributes are discussed in the final part of the chapter.

Types of information

The information, facts or evidence collected by carrying out empirical research is usually called *data*. These data (note that it is a plural noun) are often divided into two types: *hard* and *soft*. Hard data are information that can be quantified – for example, how many deaths occurred in a certain area, or how many children under five have decayed teeth? These data can be analysed using various mathematical or statistical techniques. Soft data, on the other hand, are about impressions, feelings or observations that cannot be counted – they are qualitative. Examples of qualitative data include descriptive accounts of what it is like to live in a particular area, a photographic study of a community or a video study of the elderly.

You are likely to find that these two methodological approaches are often portrayed as opposing camps, with individual sociologists positioning themselves and being categorized as 'qualitative' or 'quantitative'. This conflict is often expressed in terms of how we see the social world – 'it is measurable and can be counted' (*quantitative*) versus 'it is subjective and negotiated, and is about meanings, understandings and interpretations that cannot be counted' (*qualitative*). This distinction has often been exaggerated and has resulted in a great deal of empty posturing. The position taken in this book is a pragmatic one: 'It all depends upon what you are trying to do' (Silverman, 1997: 14).

Actual examples of these two types of data, taken from research undertaken by Bowling, are shown in Table 3.1. Both types of data are equally valid if they are appropriate to the research topic and are especially useful when used together. Examples of studies that have used both include Bowling's (1993) study of health priorities for City and Hackney Health Authority; the Kirkstall (Leeds) Local Needs survey (Percy-Smith and Sanderson, 1992); the Winnall (Winchester) project (1993); and the evaluation of the Drumchapel health project (McGhee and McEwen, 1993).

In addition to hard and soft data, information is often divided into *primary* and *secondary* data. Primary data are collected for a particular research project. For instance, the data shown in Table 3.1 were collected specifically for Bowling's study of health priorities. In contrast, secondary data are data that already exist. Hence, the data in Table 3.1 are secondary data for us. Existing data provide valuable information and should be used in all projects as a preliminary method. Studies can also be carried out by analysing these data alone. For example, many of the studies of poverty and deprivation, and the annual reports of Directors of Public Health, are produced using only secondary data (see, for instance, Abbott et al., 1992; Department of the Environment, 1995; Payne, 1995).

Table 3.1   *Examples of qualitative and quantitative data*

Qualitative data
A quotation from a depth interview

Respondent:
Prevention is better than cure. It makes more sense and, in the long run, it's cheaper to prevent people from becoming ill than treating people when they become ill. It sounds really stupid to put health education services as high until you realize that this is the thing that can stop people becoming ill in the first place.

Quantitative data
A summary from the answers to a standardized questionnaire

Health education services were ranked 14th out of 16 by the public in a priority ranking of health services.

Source: Bowling, 1993: 78, 36

All quantitative data and some qualitative data are divided into *variables*. A variable is an attribute, category or concept that can take at least two values: for example, gender (female, male); age (0 to 100 plus); and education (primary to higher). When we analyse our data we attempt to describe or discover relationships between variables. To do this we must *measure* them – give them values or categorize them in some way. In quantitative investigations this usually means assigning numeric values, while qualitative research is less involved with measurement, being usually concerned with allocating labels or categories, classifying and giving detailed descriptions.

The levels of measurement that are used to categorize variables determine the type of analysis that can be undertaken. Statisticians have classified measurement into four different levels or scales: *nominal*, *ordinal*, *interval* and *ratio*. *Nominal* measurements are those that classify things into different categories and have no numeric significance. Thus, they cannot be ranked, added, subtracted, multiplied or divided. For example, classifying patients according to in-patient or out-patient or surgical category is a nominal scale of measurement. Even if numeric categories are allocated to them for processing purposes (1 = in-patient; 2 = out-patient), these values cannot be manipulated mathematically. In-patients are neither better than, nor half the value of, out-patients. Analysis of this type of variable usually takes the form of simple *frequency distributions* (counts) such as 'the study consisted of 50 in-patients and 100 out-patients'.

The second level of measurement is *ordinal*. This scale is closer to a 'real' mathematical value than the nominal scale. Here, variables are categorized and *ranked* in some way – they are *ordered*. Like nominal scales, the ordinal level of measurement cannot be manipulated mathematically, although there is now some sequential pattern. This ranking does not, however, imply a similar numeric value between the different categories. They cannot be added, subtracted, multiplied or divided. For instance, 'upper', 'middle' and 'lower' social class and the Registrar-General's Social Classes I to V are ordinal level measurements. Social Class I is not one-fifth of Social Class V, and Social Class I plus Social Class II does not equal Social Class III.

In contrast, *interval* level measurements do have equal intervals between each category, and they can thus be ranked, added and subtracted. However, they do not have a true mathematical zero and cannot be multiplied or divided. The most frequently used example of this level of measurement are IQ scores and temperature scales. Here, we can say that a person with an IQ of 100 scores fifty points higher than one with an IQ of 50 but is not necessarily twice as intelligent.

The final measurement level, the *ratio* scale, is a full mathematical measurement with a true zero. Variables of this type can thus be ranked, added, subtracted, multiplied and divided. Examples of such scales include population size, number of houses and income. Here, £2,000 is less than £3,000, and £3,000 is less than £4,000 – the scale can be ordered. £2,000 is also £1,000 less than £3,000, and £3,000 is £1,000 less than £4,000 – the scale has equal intervals. However, with this type of measurement it is possible to say that £2,000 is two-thirds of £3,000 and half of £4,000 – it is a ratio scale.

An understanding of how variables are measured is an important factor in deciding what methods you will use to collect information, and the type of analysis that can be undertaken on the resulting data. Statistical techniques that have been devised for one level of measurement cannot be used on variables that have a lower order of measurement. These techniques will be described in Chapter 9.

Selecting information

Before collecting data, we need to decide what categories of information are relevant to our study, and from whom we are going to collect it. Categorizing information requirements involves drawing up a list of the topics or areas that we are interested in, such as housing, environment, crime. These topics are then further refined to produce a list of questions. The construction of these lists is discussed in Chapters 2 and 6.

Deciding on where and from whom to collect information is determined by the nature of your study and the resources that you have available. While it would be possible to collect information from everyone in a community, it is often not feasible nor is it necessary. Financial, personnel and time constraints mean that you will usually only be able to obtain information from some of the people you are interested in (your *population*) and you will, therefore, have to be selective.

Selecting (or *sampling*) involves making sure that you choose suitable people for your study. This means that you need to ensure that the people you select will be able to provide you with relevant information. For example, you would be unlikely to ask a sample of older people to provide you with information about child care facilities. Further, if you want to make general statements about a community, you will need to make sure that the people you select are *representative* of the people who live there. Finally, if you plan to carry out statistical analysis of the resulting data, you will need to ensure that this representative sample has been selected *randomly*. Methods of sampling are discussed in Chapter 5.

Methods of collecting information

The range and type of information that you decide to collect determines the research techniques that you need to use. For example, using existing quantitative sources (official statistics, etc.) requires skills in using libraries, computers and elementary statistical analysis, in addition to the more general evaluative and interpretative skills. These, and skills needed in the use of other secondary sources, are discussed in Chapter 4. An overview of the main methods of collecting primary information is given here. Do not worry if you do not know what the technical terms – shown in italics – mean at this stage. More detailed descriptions of particular techniques and skills are given in the following chapters.

Quantitative information is collected using standardized survey methods. For these you may have to design *questionnaires* or *interview schedules* and learn about *interviewing* procedures. The information that you collect will need to be processed using a standardized *coding scheme* and, probably, the use of a computer *spreadsheet* package. The resulting data will then be analysed using *statistical* techniques.

An alternative to designing your own questionnaire is to use an existing package. Numerous health questionnaires have been developed (see, for instance, Bowling, 1995, 1997), of which the most widely used in the UK are the *Nottingham Health Profile* and *Short Form-36* (*SF-36*). These, however, all draw on a narrow disease-based definition of health (where health is defined as the absence of illness or impairment) and are of limited use when undertaking a broader study. Other more general packages and approaches include *Compass* and *Priority Search*, but both require some preliminary research (*discussion groups* etc.) before the questions to be included are decided.

Qualitative methods call for a wide range of skills, including *non-directive* and *depth* interviewing, *group discussion* techniques and skills in *observational* methods (for example, *facilitator* skills, note taking, use of a recorder, video, photography). Processing the resulting information is often very time consuming and difficult. All of the verbal information has to be written down (*transcribed*), either at the time or from a recording, and the resulting text will then have to be *categorized* and *analysed*. Although at first sight qualitative research looks easier and friendlier for non-experts to do than quantitative research, this is not always the case. It generally takes up a lot of time and it is recommended that only experienced researchers should undertake much of this type of research. Further, if you want a video or photographic presentation to have maximum impact, it is advisable to seek help from someone with experience in these techniques.

None of the available approaches and packages is designed for qualitative projects. *Rapid Appraisal*, a 'methodology' that is gaining popularity, is really a 'mixed-method' approach – based on what Denzin

(1970) termed *data triangulation*. Using multiple methods has been common in social research for many years (for example, the Institute of Community Studies' work in the East End during the 1950s and 1960s). Although the techniques employed in *Rapid Appraisal* are not new, it does provide a framework to guide a health needs assessment by indicating the broad areas on which to concentrate. However, by limiting the questioning to prominent or 'key' people in the community, it is open to criticism regarding representativeness and bias (see Bowling, 1993; NHS Management Executive, 1992; and Chapter 8 below).

What methods to select

All of the methods discussed here have their advantages and disadvantages. Quantitative data from surveys are easier to analyse than qualitative information – if you have the necessary computing and statistical skills. However, using *rich* or qualitative data may be a better way of illustrating particular points. You need to decide what methods are the most *appropriate* or *applicable* for your study.

The choice of methods will be determined by what you want to achieve (your aims and objectives) and your financial, people and time resources. If your aim is to improve or change service provision, the socio-economic environment and/or to get more resources for a community, your evidence must be convincing and persuasive. It is more likely that you will be listened to and your arguments accepted if you base your case on information obtained using tried and tested techniques. Further, most statutory agencies need evidence to be representative of the whole community. They will want to know from whom you obtained your information and how; what questions were asked, and what is the likelihood of its being accurate. In short, they usually want a survey. This is not to say that evidence from other methods is likely to be discounted, but ideally these should be representative and be backed up by a survey.

Ideally, the best way of undertaking a community health profile or health needs assessment is to use a mixed-method approach. However, this is likely to be very expensive and you will probably have to make a compromise between your ideal methods and your resources. All of the methods of collecting information will involve some expenditure, as discussed in Chapter 2. This expenditure will range from the telephone, postage and stationery costs involved in obtaining existing information to the many resource requirements of depth interviewing and group discussions. In addition, you will need to budget for some consumables (paper etc.) used in processing and analysing your data and for your presentations.

Preliminary information

Whatever the focus of your study, it is important to carry out a thorough review of existing information. This could save you considerable time by not having to collect new information and avoid the danger of 're-inventing the wheel'. It can also act as a guide to the approach that you might adopt and forewarn you of any pitfalls. In addition to making the maximum use of existing information, it is recommended that the preliminary stage of your project should include a series of informal discussions with groups or individuals. These will enable you to have an idea about the possible range of topics to be covered and the strength of feeling about them. Sources of existing information and people to contact are discussed in Chapter 4.

Interest-based communities

Interest-based communities consist of people who share a common interest, gender, ethnicity or other characteristic. They are not necess-arily located in a particular place. These would include women, the elderly, a minority ethnic group or a church congregation, sports or social club, for example. The main problem associated with studying these groups is that of identification. Although some existing statistics are sub-divided by age, gender and ethnicity, they are very limited. If the community that you are interested in is not based on any of these broad categories, you are unlikely to find any existing statistical infor-mation. You should, however, attempt to get information on the general population so that you can make comparisons with your results. Exist-ing information may be available from studies already undertaken and it is worth spending time finding these.

When you come to collect new information, you are likely to face a second identification problem: that of obtaining a name and address list. Unless your group is one that has a list of members, you will have to decide on a way of making contact. This might be through adver-tisements or a public meeting, contacting existing organizations that might have information, or by undertaking a preliminary 'search survey' of an area.

In selecting the methods to use to get information from such groups, you should aim to include a representative cross-section of opinions. This does not necessarily mean that you will have to do a survey. For group discussions or depth interviewing, for instance, you should try to ensure that these do not just include 'activists' or your friends. The recommended methods for studying these communities are group discussions and/or surveys. For groups with a strongly committed membership, a self-completion questionnaire could be used.

Institution and work-based communities

Unlike interest-based communities, institution-based groups are always located in a particular place for a certain amount of time. These communities will include workplaces, schools, colleges or universities and residential homes/establishments. If the group that you are interested in falls into this category, you are lucky: you already have a 'captive' community and you are likely to have a list of names.

Existing information is likely to include various records that are kept for administrative purposes. However, do not assume that you will be able to access these: they are confidential and you will need permission. Alternatively, the person or department responsible for holding them may be able to give you information about the age, gender, occupation, sickness and other characteristics of the group without identifying the names of the individuals who make up the group.

The methods of collecting new information will be determined by the particular nature of the community and your position in it. For example, elderly people living in a residential home may have sight problems that might make it difficult to fill in a self-completion questionnaire. Further, employees may be reluctant to give negative information about their employers if they think that they may be identified. However, all such communities do give the opportunity for carrying out detailed observations.

Group discussions would be an appropriate method for all of these communities. However, some people may not volunteer some of their views because they can be identified by others in the group. In residential homes, individual information could be collected by one-to-one interviews, whereas in a work-based group a self-completion questionnaire could be used. Communities that are based on schools offer the widest opportunities for a mixed-method approach – but remember that researching the under-18s requires the permission of parents or guardians. Here, you could use class discussions and projects, augmented by a one-to-one interview survey designed for particular age groups.

Locality-based communities

These groups are what we usually think of when we talk about 'communities'. They are people who live in a particular geographical area.

Locality-based communities usually include many of the previous two types. Thus any of the methods suggested as being suitable for interest and institutional-based communities can be used. For a general study of the health needs of a locality-based community a combination of observation and *Rapid Appraisal* techniques are recommended as a first stage. However, because of the limitations of *Rapid Appraisal* (especially the reliance on 'key informants'), these methods should be backed up by a series of group discussions and a community survey.

Validity and reliability

In addition to being appropriate to our research, methods of collecting information need to be *valid* and *reliable*. These two interrelated concepts refer to the confidence that is given to the resulting findings: a valid and reliable method should produce valid and reliable data. *Validity* is about whether the techniques used *measure what they are meant to* – that they will produce accurate findings. *Reliability* is concerned with whether the techniques *produce data that are consistent* – when repeated they will produce similar findings. Thus, although a valid method is usually reliable, it does not necessarily follow that a reliable method is valid. In quantitative research, and particularly in health-related measures, much greater emphasis has been placed on validity and reliability testing than in more qualitative studies. This emphasis is sometimes so great that descriptions of the methods themselves appear to be much shorter than descriptions of their validation and reliability (for example, Bowling, 1995, 1997).

Validity

In textbooks you will often come across terms such as *content validity*, *face validity*, *criterion validity*, *concurrent validity* and *predictive validity*. For your purposes – and, perhaps, for the sake of your sanity – it is not necessary to distinguish between the particular semantic differences. Basically, there are two types of validity: *empirical* and *theoretical*. In tests of empirical validity, the technique is valid if it produces results that are consistent with existing and future findings from other studies. Theoretical validity, on the other hand, is concerned with whether the technique is consistent with existing theoretical and common sense understandings. For instance, a study that found that there were significantly higher rates of ill health in an affluent area than in a poor one might not be seen as valid, either theoretically or empirically. In this case, we would examine the definitions and operational measures of 'ill health', 'affluence' and 'poverty', and the selection processes used in the study.

Reliability

As with validity tests, you will sometimes read about the *test–retest* method, the *split half* method, the *multiple form* method and *inter-item* tests. Here again, you should not worry about these terms. Reliability tests are concerned with repeatability or consistency. These methods test for consistency over time, between different groups and internal to the method itself. For example, asking a person's date of birth is more reliable over time and between groups than asking for their age. Again, if you are concerned with life histories, you should use either dates or ages throughout the study rather than mixing them. Although, here, mixed-methods could be used for internal checking.

You should not worry too much about the various tests for validity and reliability that might be undertaken. What really matters is whether the methods used actually work and are *appropriate* for your study. If you are worried, you should talk to your tutor or a social research expert. Those trained in the more 'positivist' sciences such as medicine and psychology are likely to be more concerned about validity and reliability tests than those from a sociology, social policy or community work background.

Alternative perspectives

Questions about whether scientifically valid, reliable and objective methods are possible in research have been issues of debate since the Enlightenment. More recently, theoretical developments (for instance, chaos theory, postmodernism) have raised further doubts about these concepts. In qualitative social research, especially, both the presence of a researcher and the research act itself are thought to bring about changes in what people say and do that make traditional scientific replication and verification unattainable. Instead, terms such as 'trustworthy', 'dependable', 'legitimate' and 'credible' research have been advanced. The principle technique for achieving these goals is through *reflexive subjectivity*. Here, researchers include, as part of their research, a consideration of how their personal thoughts, feelings, experiences, actions and beliefs impact upon the research process. These are recorded in a research diary or journal. A full discussion of these issues is given in Grbich, (1999: 13–24, 58–80). However, inexperienced researchers have sometimes become more interested in introspection than in getting the research done. It is also worth remembering that a final report will have more **political** impact if it is not overloaded with self-reflection, doubts and personal considerations.

Chapter summary

Empirical research involves collecting information is a systematic way so that findings are justifiable and credible. This chapter has examined the types of information (*data*) that might be collected, and how these can be classified or *measured*: *quantitatively* and *qualitatively*. Data are available at different *levels of measurement*. The methods for doing this are by reading, asking questions and observing.

All research involves reading and using *existing information*, and in some projects this is the only method used. However, usually we find that we need to collect new data. These are obtained using structured *survey* techniques or more detailed *depth interviewing*, including *group discussions*. *Observational* methods are used to record events as they happen. They can be structured and quantifiable or more descriptive accounts of social interactions. Often a *mixed-method* strategy is adopted. This allows for data corroboration (*triangulation*) and for the collection of a wider range of data.

Whatever methods are selected, it is important that they should be appropriate to your study. If you want to find out how many people have been hospital in-patients during the past year, a study using observational or depth interviewing techniques would be unsuitable. Equally, if you intend to investigate interactions between staff and patients in a hospital, it is unlikely that you would use health authority statistical data or survey a sample of the general public. The methods used and your resulting evidence are expected to be *valid* and *reliable*.

Exercise

1   List five examples for each of the following levels of measurement:

    (a) nominal
    (b) ordinal
    (c) interval
    (d) ratio

2   Discuss the validity of studies devised to examine traffic flow in a city by:

    (a) Counting traffic entering the city from the north at 11 a.m. on a Sunday
    (b) a survey about car ownership from a sample of addresses in the city
    (c) analysing the number of parking spaces in the central area of the city

---

CHAPTER 4

USING EXISTING INFORMATION

Once you have decided on the information that you need to meet the aims and objectives of your project, the next step should be to discover how much of this information is already available. You may think that there is little or no existing information available on the topic that concerns you, but this is highly unlikely. People do not usually volunteer information unless asked, and public agencies do not usually share information or advertise the fact that they hold a range of information. This is not necessarily because they are being awkward or secretive but because communicating information is not central to their main function. You should therefore try to find out about all possible sources. Using existing information is a relatively cheap and quick way of getting an overall picture of a community and, in some cases, may provide you with all the information that you require.

In this chapter we will examine the main sources of existing information. First, we will discuss what we mean by 'existing' information and how it has been used. However, because this information is, by definition, collected for other purposes, it is important that anyone using existing sources is aware of their limitations, validity and reliability. We will then look at ways to find out about what information is readily accessible and how to access it. The main national and local sources are then described, along with the most widely used deprivation indices. Finally, the chapter gives guidance on how these data might be used in your own research projects.

What is existing information?

Existing information or 'secondary data' comes in many forms. These range from the statistical (numerical) reports produced by central government departments, local councils and health authorities to small scale community studies undertaken by, for example, voluntary organizations, university researchers or school projects. Additionally, local newspapers may have done special reports or someone may have produced a video or photographic study. An organization's staff or membership records would also come into this category, although it is likely that the information would need further processing (and, in such cases, the principle of informed consent should be adhered to). It is worth spending some time in tracking down all of these various sources before embarking on any new data collection.

Even if existing sources do not provide you with all of the information that you need, they can be used as important preliminary sources of data, as complementary to your project or to compare your study with others. For example, the Winall survey, discussed in Chapter 2, looked at local statistics from the 1991 Census and three previous local studies before collecting new information. The *Rapid Appraisal* method, to be discussed in Chapter 8, uses existing information to complement and substantiate findings from other techniques, and information from the 1991 Population Census was used to investigate poverty, health and social class in Devon and Cornwall (Payne, G. et al., 1996; Payne, J. et al., 1996).

The limitations of existing information

When using existing information sources it is important to be aware of their limitations. Of particular importance are geographical coverage, timeliness, completeness and the original source. In statistical sources, geographical coverage and definitional changes over time can be especially problematic.

For administrative purposes, the United Kingdom of Great Britain and Northern Ireland is divided *geographically* into eleven Standard Regions. These are Northern Ireland, Scotland, Wales, North, North West, Yorkshire and Humberside, East Midlands, West Midlands, East Anglia, South East and South West. These regions are then divided into Counties, then Districts (coinciding with local authority District Councils). Some large urban areas are designated 'unitary authorities' which replace the County/District division. These are further divided into wards for electoral and census purposes. The Census of Population also uses smaller area units called 'enumeration districts' that comprise about 200 households. Other agencies are increasingly using post codes instead of enumeration districts. Post codes were used in Scotland for the 1991 Population Census and will also be used in England and Wales for the 2001 Census.

Health Authority, Social Services and Police Authority boundaries do not necessarily coincide with any or all of these. In Devon, an area familiar to the author, the South and West Devon Health Authority consists of the unitary authorities of Plymouth and Torbay, the Districts of South Hams and Teignbridge, and parts of the West Devon District. In the City of Plymouth itself, different locality boundaries are used by the Police Authority, the Social Services Department, the Health Authority and the Housing Department, although attempts are being made for these to coincide. In addition to these variations, local economic data are often presented for Travel to Work Areas (TTWA) that also have different boundaries. Thus, the Plymouth TTWA consists of the City of Plymouth plus parts of the South Hams and parts of West Devon, plus parts of the Caradon District in Cornwall.

Other data are often only available at the higher geographical levels. For example, before undertaking any new data collection in the Devonport area of Plymouth, Lapthorne (1996) identified the following existing data sources: census data; mortality data; morbidity data; perinatal data; immunization rates; infectious disease notification; cancer registration; and in-patient episodes (see the Glossary for definitions). However, because these data were often only available at local authority or health district level rather than at *ward* level, their collection and processing was difficult. Data had to be extracted by hand, and reprocessed or approximations had to be made. These inconsistencies in coverage and area aggregation are found in most parts of Britain.

A further problem encountered in locality studies is that of changing definitions over *time*. These changes occur because of population changes between Population Censuses (an enumeration district is defined as the number of households that an enumerator can cover in a day). There have been, and there are likely to be future, changes in boundaries through local government reorganizations and health authority mergers, or to suit other administrative conveniences. Such changes can make comparisons over time either extremely difficult or impossible. For example, in compiling the *Index of Local Conditions* for the Department of the Environment, Robson and his colleagues had to convert the 1991 Population Census data to 1981-based wards before any comparisons could be made (Department of the Environment, 1995: 123).

In addition to these changes in boundary definitions, there are often changes in the data definitions themselves. Unemployment statistics have been particularly inconsistent, with many different measurements being used (see, for instance, Denman and McDonald, 1996). Further, households, although once defined as those sharing at least one meal per day in the Population Census, are now usually determined by enumerators (Sapsford and Abbott, 1992: 65). These are just two of many examples of changing definitions in general statistical information. In health related data, the most notable recent change was that brought about by changing estimations of fetal viability, necessitating changes in the definitions of stillbirth and abortion/miscarriage.

Other differences occur because of changes in the way in which the data are collected. Thus ethnicity was defined by asking about place of birth in the 1981 Census whereas, in 1991, this was determined by asking individuals how they defined themselves. A further limitation related to timeliness is the age of the data themselves. Here, it is important to discover when the information was collected, whether there have been significant changes since then, and if there are any alternative sources of data that could be used instead. The Population Census, one of the most useful demographic sources, is only collected every ten years and, thus, information from the last one (in 1991) is now more than eight years out of date.

Completeness can refer to either population or data coverage. For example, as we shall see in Chapter 5, surveys based on a sample drawn from telephone directories will not include those who have recently had a telephone installed, are ex-directory or who do not have a telephone. It will, however, still contain those who have died, moved away or have been disconnected for whatever reason. Missing data, on the other hand, can refer to information that people have refused to give, do not know, or that has not been asked for. Thus the 1991 Census asks about 'limiting long term illness', but does not ask about the nature of the illness and would not, therefore, be sufficient for use on its own in a health needs assessment.

A further limitation to the use of secondary information is that of the *reputation and capability* of the person or agency that produced them. This not only concerns their general research standing but also refers to the methods used to collect and analyse the data, and to any bias that they might have. Disraeli's often quoted statement about 'lies, damned lies and statistics' refers to the process by which data can sometimes be manipulated to support opposing views. Thus an agency might use one set of data showing high levels of poverty, unemployment and homelessness to support its case for additional government funding, while also using photographs of attractive environments, varied leisure activities and happy people to attract tourists to the same area.

Questions that should be asked when using existing information are shown in Table 4.1. These relate to the four potential problem areas discussed here. In addition, you should also ask general questions about validity and reliability, as discussed in Chapter 3.

Where to find out about existing information

Perhaps the best way of finding out about what information already exists is to visit your local public, university, college or school libraries. They will probably hold, or be able to obtain, copies of the most important government statistical reports and various annual and special reports undertaken by local agencies. In addition, there is likely to be a local history/studies section that may be worth examining.

The key to making the most of these library sources is to approach

Table 4.1 *Questions to ask when using existing information*

Question	Amplification
Geographical	
What geographical areas are covered?	Often health authority, local authority and police authority boundaries, for example, do not coincide
Have the boundaries changed?	If you are comparing information over time, this is very important
Timeliness	
How old is the information?	Is it up to date? Many calculations are based on data from the latest Population Census that can be ten years out of date. Are there any other sources that might be used?
Have there been any changes in the definitions used?	Many definitions change over time. For example, unemployment. This also differs between agencies
Completeness	
Is the information complete?	For example, information on household eating patterns might exclude meals eaten away from home or snacks
What information is missing?	Does it give all of the information that you need for your study?
Source and methods	
What organization has collected and processed the information?	Do they have the necessary skills? Is there any danger of bias?
What methods have been used to collect and analyse the data?	Are they valid, reliable and appropriate?
Do the results meet the aims and objectives of the project?	Does it achieve what it set out to achieve?
Are the findings consistent with the information presented?	Do you reach the same conclusions?

Source: Adapted from Hawtin, Hughes and Percy-Smith, 1994

the local librarian for help. Because of their knowledge of their library and their specialist training, librarians will probably be able to provide you with the information that you require far more quickly than if you tried to track it down yourself. Remember that part of a librarian's job is to assist you in finding relevant information.

Other sources of local information are the research and information departments of local authorities, health authorities, the various health trusts and Community Health Councils. In addition, the major voluntary organizations (for example, Citizens Advice Bureaux) and Local

Training and Enterprise Councils are likely to hold information relevant to their organizational needs. Local MPs and councillors may also be able to assist. Further, GPs and health visitors may have undertaken profiles that may be of use.

An important point to remember when approaching local agencies is that the people responsible for this information are usually extremely busy. They are most likely to be cooperative if you are clear about the information that you need and what you are going to do with it. It is therefore important that you write a list of the topics that you are interested in before approaching them. This should be by letter or phone in the first instance. Some information will be confidential and you must accept that you will not be able to have access to this. An example of such a list is given in Table 4.2. Also, do not expect to obtain the information immediately, especially if you want non-routine information. However, if you have not received the information that you have asked for within a month, or two weeks later than was promised, it is worth a gentle reminder.

In addition to, or instead of, asking people for information, you should make use of the wide range of computer-based search engines available at many libraries and via the Internet. If you have access to a computer, this is probably the most efficient method of finding out about existing sources. However, it can be compulsive (and expensive if you pay the phone bills!), so it is advisable to decide what type of information you need beforehand. If you are unsure about using these facilities, you should consult a data librarian.

Most university and college libraries now have on-line catalogues that allow you to search for information in different ways: by author or by title or by *keywords*, for example. The keywords option is likely to be the most useful method in the initial stages of your search. To do this, you must first work out the particular categories or areas that you are interested in: for example, you might decide on 'statistics' and

Table 4.2 *Example of an information requirements list*

Area:	'Newcity' and 'Oldward' separately	
Information:	Population characteristics: (percentages and raw figures)	
	Age structure:	under 5s
		over 75s
		Total
	Housing:	Owner-occupiers
		Local authority/housing association
		Total
	Long term illness:	16–pension age
		Total

'health'. When you select the keyword option of the catalogue search facility, you would enter these two words separated by a space. The computer software package would then search the library database for references that match both of these words, separately and combined. It would then give you the option of viewing the list of references for each separate category (statistics, health) or for the combined category (statistics and health together). If you use broad categories like 'statistics' and 'health', it is best to choose the combined option. You might otherwise be presented with too many references to handle or select from. Alternatively, you might want to refine your search categories by adding a further category such as 'mortality' or a particular geographical location or time period. Figure 4.1 gives an example of how these searches work.

Your library might also have access to other information sources on either CD-ROM catalogues or via the Internet. Your data librarian will be able to help you with this information. CD-ROM catalogues are used in the same way as other computer CD-ROM disks. Each one will have its own query facilities, but all will be basically the same as the example shown in Figure 4.1.

When you use the Internet or, more correctly, the world wide web, you will need to use what is called a 'search engine'. There are many of these available, of which the most common are Search UK, UK Plus, UK Yellow Web and Yahoo UK in the United Kingdom. For world wide access you could use AltaVista, Excite, Infoseek, Lycos, WebCrawler or Yahoo. These use search facilities similar to the example given in Figure 4.1, but are more extensive and allow more complex searches to be undertaken. You can search these for a wide range of information that might be of use to you. However, you can spend a considerable amount of time and effort using these as direct search tools. Instead, you could use them to access the web sites of central and local government departments, health authorities and organizations, universities and other on-line gateways and indexes that are relevant to your project.

The most useful indexes for health-related information are OMNIuk or OMNIworld; BioMedLink; BUBL; Healthfinder; and Medline. In addition, SOSIG and BIDS list wider social science sources. Information about, and produced by, the Department of Health, other government departments, the World Health Organization, and individual health and local authorities can be accessed via any of the general search engines. The range of sites and information available via the world wide web is expanding at such a rate that it is difficult to provide an up to date list in a traditionally produced paper-based book. Although the most useful sites to date are given here, it is important that you seek expert help (a data librarian or your tutor, for example) when you use these on-line facilities.

SEARCH THE ON-LINE CATALOGUE

    1   Enquiry using AUTHOR with TITLE
    2   KEYWORD enquiry
    3   TITLE enquiry
    4   NAME enquiry
    5   JOURNAL title or keyword enquiry
    6   Other

Enter code: **2**

Enter brief description: **health statistics**

'health'   4000+ items found
'statistics'   1000+ items found

---

178 items match your search

    1   Display records
    2   Go back
    3   Amend or edit this search

Enter code: **3**

Enter brief description: health statistics **mortality**

'health'   4000+ items found
'statistics'   1000+ items found
'mortality'   85 items found

---

29 items match your search

    1   Display records
    2   Go back
    3   Amend or edit this search

Enter code: **3**

Enter brief description: health statistics mortality **smoking**

'health'   4000+ items found
'statistics'   1000+ items found
'mortality'   85 items found
'smoking'   80 items found

---

1 item matches your search

    1   Display records
    2   Go back
    3   Amend or edit this search

Enter code: **1**

---

    1   Mortality from smoking in developed countries, 1950–2000: indirect estimates
        from national vital statistics/Richard Peto......[et al.].......1994

        FULL, LOCATION, BACK

Enter code:

Figure 4.1 *Example of using an on-line library catalogue. Each box represents an interactive screen on a computer. **Bold** type represents user responses*

Sources of existing information

National and international statistics

By far the most detailed information available at the national, regional and local levels is the Population Census that is undertaken every 10 years. The last one was carried out in 1991 and, although this had a higher non-response rate than expected, it is still the most reliable source of demographic, social and economic information for the various geographical levels. Its main drawback is, however, that it quickly becomes dated. Information is collected from private households and communal establishments (hospitals, nursing homes, boarding schools, prisons etc.) about the characteristics of the individuals actually or usually present. Tabulations are available on a wide range of topics including age, gender and ethnic origin; occupation, industry and employment status; housing; family type and size; qualifications; car ownership and travel to work patterns; and long term illness.

Because tabulations are available for geographical areas down to the enumeration district level, they are, perhaps, the most useful source of existing information for small scale community profiling. However, it must be remembered that, for reasons of confidentiality, the tables refer to *areas* not *individuals*. You would not be able to find out, for example, how many lone parents had professional occupations, cars or were suffering from a long term illness, only how many people in each category there were in a particular area.

Other useful sources of national statistical information published annually are *Social Trends*, *Regional Trends*, *The New Earnings Survey*, *Health and Personal Social Services Statistics*, *General Household Survey*, *Family Expenditure Survey* and the *National Food Survey*. *Population Trends*, produced quarterly, provides updates on population projections and vital statistics (births and deaths). Unfortunately, few of the tables included in these publications are for area aggregates below the Standard Region or Regional Health Authority area level. Even when sub-regional tables are produced, these are usually only available for counties. *Regional Trends* does, however, include a selection of tables at the local authority district level.

All of these publications are available through local libraries. However, many national statistics are also available on computer disks (floppy or CD-ROM) or via on-line query. The main suppliers are the Office of National Statistics (ONS) via StatBase; the Economic and Social Research Council's (ESRC) Data Archive and Qualitative Data Archive at Essex University; and MIDAS at Manchester University. A good starting point for on-line enquiries about government statistical information would be the CCTA government information service at

<http://www.open.gov.uk/>. Some of these sites only provide data to bona fide researchers. In which case, you will need to complete a licence application form and possibly purchase the data sets.

A wide range of statistical information is available for comparative purposes at the international level. Of particular relevance are those produced by EUROSTAT for the European Union, the World Health Organization and the Organization for Economic Co-operation and Development (OECD). All produce statistics relating to health and social conditions on an annual basis (for example, the OECD's *Annual Health Data*). In addition, ad hoc reports are produced frequently. All of these sources are listed at the organizations' web sites on the Internet.

Local statistics

Probably the most extensive source of local statistical information will be held by your local authority. This will include information covering population, housing, employment, tourism, agriculture, environment, transport, education, social services and crime. The particular department responsible for collating this information varies between authorities. It could be 'Planning', 'Economic Development', 'Research and Intelligence' or the 'Chief Executive's Office'. Other departments such as 'Housing' and 'Environmental Health' will also hold local information relating to their specific responsibilities.

Each health authority produces an annual report by its Director of Public Health that includes a set of tables covering birth and death rates by cause, cancer registration and *Health of the Nation* monitoring information. These rates are produced for the health authority areas as a whole and are, therefore, of limited value for small locality studies. However, health authorities have 'Research and Information' departments that might be able to provide more detailed information for smaller areas. Information is also collected at the regional level.

As with national statistics, it is now increasingly common for local and health authorities to provide information about their areas of responsibility via the Internet. These can be accessed using the search facilities described earlier in this chapter. However, it is probably best to make personal contact before accessing local information because you are then most likely to be given the more detailed information that is often not provided on web pages.

Deprivation indexes

Deprivation is a term that is used to describe a relative need or a lack of social and material resources. The term is used to describe individuals and geographical areas. This definition implies that any attempts at measurement have to be made *indirectly* by measuring social or material resources. Further, although there have been numerous attempts to categorize these measures, there is no real consensus of what 'social and material resources' to measure. In 1976 the OECD produced a list of ten categories of 'social well being' (health; individual development through learning; employment and quality of life; time and leisure; personal economic situation; physical environment; social environment; personal safety and administration of justice; social opportunity and participation; accessibility) but gave no indication of how to define and measure these various dimensions. For example, how do you measure 'health' or 'quality of life'? For a full discussion of these issues see Department of the Environment (1995).

Studies of deprivation have therefore had to use a range of indicators as proxies for these dimensions. For instance, home ownership is often used as an indicator of wealth and car ownership as an indicator of income. The measurements of each indicator have then been added together to form indexes of deprivation. Thus indexes of deprivation are attempts to combine the various dimensions into a single multi-dimensional score. For a more detailed discussion of the problems associated with measuring deprivation, and for descriptions of the statistical techniques used, see Department of the Environment (1995) and Payne (1995).

The close association established between deprivation and poor health (Department of Health, 1998b; Townsend et al., 1992) has led to the use of these indexes in studies of health needs to both compare areas and to determine 'at risk' localities. The most widely used of these are the Jarman Underprivileged Area Scores (UPA) developed in 1983; the Townsend Material Deprivation Index; and the Index of Local Conditions (ILC) and its update, the Index of Local Deprivation (ILD). There have been many criticisms of each of these indexes, and all have advantages and disadvantages. However, although they are based on different indicators and different scoring systems, they show very similar patterns in the distribution of deprivation. With the exception of the ILD, the indexes are based primarily on census data and thus measure area rather than individual deprivation.

The *UPA* was constructed as a method of assessing the workload of GPs in response to reports that drew attention to geographical variations in the demand for primary care (Jarman, 1983). Eight census area indicators were selected from an initial list of twenty-one possible measurements. These were: unemployment; overcrowding; low social class; lone parent households; lone pensioner households; children under the age of 5; movers; those born in the New Commonwealth. These indicators were subject to statistical transformation before being added together to give a score for each census ward. Although the UPA was designed primarily to guide the allocation of additional allowances to GPs, it has been used in many health related studies as a deprivation measure (see, for instance, Department of Health, 1998a, 1998b). The UPA scores can be obtained from your local health authority.

Townsend's index was developed after extensive research into poverty and deprivation in London, Bristol and the North of England (Townsend et al., 1988). This index is an attempt to identify *material* deprivation by using four census variables: unemployment; over-crowding; non-owner-occupier households; no car households. These measurements are first transformed statistically before being added to give an overall score for each area. Despite using only four variables, the Townsend index is widely acknowledged to be the best index of material deprivation currently available. Morris and Carstairs (1991) found it to have the highest correlation with other indexes and the best predictor of premature death. Scores on this index are given for each local authority in England in Gordon and Forrest (1995).

The *Index of Local Conditions* (Department of the Environment, 1995) was developed as a replacement for the earlier Index of Urban Depri-vation (Department of the Environment, 1983). The Index attempts to combine variables from the 1991 Population Census with other measures to produce scores that can be applied at the local authority district, ward and enumeration district levels. The seven census vari-ables used were: unemployment; overcrowding; lack of basic ameni-ties; no car households; children living in unsuitable accommodation; children in low earning households; 17-year-olds not in full time edu-cation. In addition, six non-census variables were used at the local authority district level. These were: Standard Mortality Ratio (SMR); long term unemployed; income support recipients; house content insurance premiums; low GCSE attainment; amount of derelict land. Again, these were statistically transformed and added to give a total score. Because the ILC was used in the allocation of regeneration grants, it was criticized by many, particularly rural, local authorities on the basis of the variables selected and the use of out of date census vari-ables.

Its replacement, the 1998 *Index of Local Deprivation* (Department of the Environment, Transport and the Regions, 1998) includes updated figures where possible, drops 'children in unsuitable accommodation' and car ownership, and replaces the 1991 Census unemployment rate with a 1997 rate. The 1991 Census-derived variable 'children in low earning households' is replaced by 1996 Department of Social Security data on dependent children of income support recipients, and a new variable from the same source, 'non income support recipients in receipt of council tax benefit' replaces the car ownership variable. This index has only been in operation since April 1998 and it is therefore too early to assess its validity and reliability. It does, however, have the advantage of timeliness that the other indexes lack. Scores for all local authorities in England are given in Department of the Environment (1995) and Department of the Environment, Transport and the Regions (1998).

Existing research studies

A considerable amount of research has been carried out on the health profiles of communities. These studies have used many different methods of collecting information, ranging from the highly statistical to the more qualitative methods of community research. Many have used a multi-method approach. Such research should be consulted both for examples of these methods and for their findings. Some of the most useful studies are discussed here.

The most recent extensive review of health in England is the Department of Health's *Inquiry into Inequalities in Health* (1998b). Before this, the most important national reports were *The Black Report* (Townsend and Davidson, 1982) and *The Health Divide* (Whitehead, 1988). These are published and updated in Townsend et al. (1992). All of these studies show that inequalities in the health status of the poorest and wealthiest social groups still exist fifty years after the NHS was founded and have, if anything, widened over the past decade.

Since the earlier reports were published a large number of studies have been undertaken illustrating various aspects of the link between poverty and ill-health in many different locations. The main findings of these studies are discussed in Benzeval et al. (1995) and Laughlin and Black (1995). Studies showing the widening gap in health status between 1981 and 1991 include those carried out in Glasgow by McLoone and Boddy (1994) and in Middlesborough by Phillimore et al. (1994).

Since the changes in the NHS after the 1990 Act (for example, the introduction of an internal market, emphasis on primary and community care etc.) and the NHS Management Executive's guidance for local consultations in 1992 (*Local Voices*), numerous projects have been undertaken by many different groups and agencies. These include those carried out by local health authorities themselves (for example, Calderdale and Kirklees, Somerset, City and Hackney), GP/health visitor studies (for instance, Isle of Wight, Dumbiedykes) and many *Healthy Cities* initiatives in Sheffield, Leeds, Liverpool, Glasgow, Hull and Camden. Before undertaking new research it is essential to read some of the reports from these studies for ideas and possible frameworks on which to base your project.

The interpretation of existing information

It is clear from the previous descriptions that existing information comes in many forms. It might be quantitative, as raw or processed data, or it might be more qualitative in the form of textual or visual descriptions, or it might be a mixture of both. However, it is unlikely that it will be in the exact format that you need. Once you have decided that the information is applicable to your study and that it is valid and reliable, you will need to select the parts that are relevant for your purpose. You should also bear in mind copyright restrictions (including photocopying), and always reference your sources.

Usually, official statistics such as those produced in *Regional Trends* or census reports are presented as large, detailed tables in a format similar to that given in Table 4.3. Here you would select out the variables that you are interested in for your area, and for other areas with which you might want to make comparisons. The data may be presented as counts (as would be the case in Table 4.3), percentages, or rates and ratios. It is therefore important to discover the units of measurement used and the time period covered before you undertake any detailed analysis yourself.

Health related data are often presented as rates, ratios and risk levels, such as the Standard Mortality Ratio (SMR). These and other epidemiological terms are defined in the Glossary. Here again, it is important to establish the population base and the units of measurement used before undertaking any further analysis or using them as evidence.

In both quantitative and qualitative research reports you should find out what methods were used to obtain the information presented and discover what population was covered. Again, you should scrutinize the reports using the questions discussed earlier in this chapter and shown in Table 4.1. Further detailed guidance on assessing such reports is given in Sapsford and Abbott (1992: 19–75).

Once assessed for applicability, reliability and validity, secondary data are analysed using similar methods to those used in the analysis of new data. These are discussed in Chapters 9 and 10.

Chapter summary

Before collecting new information you should attempt to discover what information already exists about your research topic. This information is mainly in the form of *statistics*, *reports* and findings from *other studies*. These are available for various geographical areas from the international to the very local.

Table 4.3 *Example of existing statistical information*

	Area (sq km)	Persons (per sq km)	Population (thousands)			Total Population percentage change 19xx–19xx	Total Period Fertility Rate (TPFR)	Standardized Mortality Ratio (SMR)
			Males	Females	Total			
United Kingdom	*	*	*	*	*	*	*	*
Region	*	*	*	*	*	*	*	*
County	*	*	*	*	*	*	*	*
District	*	*	*	*	*	*	*	*

Note: actual names would replace the Region, County and District, and * would be replaced by actual counts and rates.
Source: adapted from *Regional Trends*, Table 15.1

This chapter has discussed the major sources of this information in relation to coverage, limitations, validity and reliability. Getting hold of information involves finding out who has it, and then asking for it in a specific way. Not all available information will be in a form suitable for you to use. Some information is confidential, and you may be refused access. Besides asking, you should familiarize yourself with *library catalogue search techniques*. Recently, a wide range of information has become available through the *Internet*. Although the main web sites have been mentioned here, the *world wide web* is expanding so fast that many other sites will be on-line before this book is published.

Exercise

Assess the applicability, reliability and validity of any *one* of the existing sources mentioned in this chapter or listed in the Case Studies at the end of the book.

CHAPTER 5

SELECTING RESPONDENTS

For any research that involves the collection of new information, you will need to decide from which people to collect it. This means that, at the outset, you must *define the population* that you are interested in so that you can select from it. The resources (time, money, personnel, expertise) you have available and the type of information that you want to collect do, of course, influence how you make your selection. However, your knowledge of the people you are interested in is of primary importance.

It is often assumed that systematic methods of selecting respondents are only used in quantitative (survey) research, and that they are not necessary for the less structured methods of qualitative research. This assumption is mistaken, since the way in which you select your respondents is important in determining the validity and reliability of your study whatever approach you adopt.

In this chapter we will look at the ways in which you might go about choosing who you will get data from – your population *units*; whether to select everyone or just some – a *census* or a *sample*; and the most common methods of sampling.

Defining your population

In a strictly statistical sense, a *population* can refer to a group of any type of unit: widgets, trees, atoms and so on. In social research, these units are either individual people or collections of people. The population that you are interested in will either be a locality-based or an interest-based community, and you are likely to refer to it in these terms: Lower Downs Estate, sixth formers at Blankton School, or mothers and toddlers, for example. Such terms, although useful labels in general conversation, do not provide a precise enough definition for selection purposes. In the type of research that you will be undertaking, your population will be defined in terms of location, time, attribute, or all three. Thus, Blankton School is a *location*, and the sixth formers are those in a particular age group (*attribute*) at a particular *time*.

In defining a locality-based population, you will need to decide on the exact geographical boundaries of the community, and whether to include only those who live there or others who work there or are political representatives, visitors etc. In these situations, it is worth walking around the locality, preferably with a large scale map, to decide what streets are to be included. Further, for those streets that are to be boundaries, you will have to decide whether both sides or only one are in your population. If you decide to include people who work in the locality, you will need to list all the relevant groups. These will include local authority and health workers, shopkeepers and publicans, solicitors, police, voluntary organizations, delivery and other personal service providers, local councillors, MPs and religious leaders. These processes should be undertaken for any location, even if it is familiar. However well we think that we know an area, there are always some parts (and people) with which we are unfamiliar.

Institution-based communities might be seen as more easily defined. Here, your population will be those who attend, work or live in particular buildings or institutions. In addition, you will have to decide whether to include other people who may be of interest. For example, family members may provide relevant information and, when studying under-18-year-olds, parents or guardians should be informed. Further, the time period for inclusion should be clearly defined. This is particularly important in those institutions in which there is a fairly rapidly changing population such as hospitals, clubs and playgroups. In such instances, you might decide to include all of those who attend during your field work phase or you might include those who have attended since a particular date. This latter method was used by Abbott and Payne (1992) in their study of open-heart surgery patients where they selected patients from both the previous and current year.

Interest-based communities have different definitional problems from those discussed above. Here membership is not necessarily constrained by geographical boundaries. The health needs of women, for example, could require an international study involving historical and current research. However, it is more likely that you will confine your study to a particular locality and time. If you make such selections, you should be careful when making any generalizations, since your particular population may not be representative of the wider interest group.

In addition to this broad population definition, you will need to decide whether you want to collect information about individuals or groups – your *population units*. Our previous example on the health needs of women can be used to illustrate this choice. Here you may decide to include in your population all women over 18 years of age in a particular locality. Alternatively, you may define your population as households in particular localities or women's organizations in particular localities. In the first instance your population units would be women, in the second, households and, in the third, women's organizations. Clearly, the type of questions you would ask and the information you would obtain are likely to differ according to the unit selected. Your choice would be determined by the nature of your research, your particular perspective, and your resources.

Population lists

Once you have defined exactly who you are interested in, you will need to know whether you have, or can compile, a list of everybody in your chosen population. If you have, or can draw up, a list, you can select from it, otherwise you will have to use another method such as the ones discussed later (*quota sampling* or *snowballing*, for example).

There are many different sources of population lists. These include membership lists, electoral registers, council tax lists, GP patient lists and telephone directories, or you might collect addresses of all the residential dwellings in a particular area. The main requirements of such lists are that they should be as *up to date*, *complete*, *accurate* and *suitable* as possible. In addition, if you are only going to select some people, the list should also be ordered in such a way that everyone on it has a known chance of being selected. Thus, there should be no grouping by attributes such as age, gender or ethnicity, and there should be no duplication.

For example, a two-year-old telephone directory would not be *up to date* and would therefore include people who had left the area or had died, and would exclude newcomers. Further, not everyone has a telephone and some people are ex-directory: it would not be *complete*. It might also include people who had moved address or changed their name but had retained their telephone number, or those who had taken over someone else's number: it would not be *accurate*. Also, it would not be *suitable* for surveys of certain groups: women, pensioners, etc. Very few lists are perfect and often one has to make use of the best available. Government social surveys now often use post codes and house numbers to get around these problems – housing does not change as much as people do.

Census or sample

If you have a suitable list of your population, you then have to decide whether to select all of those on the list (a *census*) or just a few (a *sample*). The term 'census' is often confused with the Census of Population that is undertaken every ten years in the UK. This is just a well-known example of a census, which simply means the collection of information from/about each population unit. Collecting information in this way will certainly give you a complete account, but it can be extremely expensive and time consuming.

Unless your community is very small, it is neither possible nor necessary to get information from every single person in it. What you need is a *sample*: a selection from the *population*. A sample is a smaller sub-set of all the possible people who might be included. If it is a properly selected sample it will be representative of the total population of people (or households) who make up your community. Sample size is discussed later in this chapter.

The best way to get a representative sample is to pick people or households in a way that prevents the person doing the selection having any say in who gets drawn, rather like the National Lottery draw. This is called *random* sampling, the word 'random' being a technical term meaning that the selection is not biased to over-represent any one group. Sometimes random sampling is referred to as *probability* sampling. This is because, in the process of selection, everyone has an equal (in simple random sampling) or known (in stratified sampling) *chance* or *probability* of being selected. If you are undertaking quantitative research, provided you have a random sample, it is possible to do statistical analysis on the data you collect.

The overall answers you obtain from a good sample will be very close indeed to the answers you would have obtained if you had questioned everybody. It is true that the sample's answers are only estimates, and you need to remember this in reporting what you find out. However, if all aspects of the research are properly carried out, the estimates based on the sample will be very close to what the whole population would say. With a random sample, you can calculate just how close by using *confidence levels*: research reports sometimes say things like 'The proportion saying they visited their GP in the last year was 45 per cent, plus or minus 2 per cent'. What this means is that the researchers know that 45 per cent of the *sample* did it, and it can be estimated that between 43 per cent and 47 per cent of the *population* did it. Confidence levels are discussed in Chapter 9.

The key requirement of your sample is that it is *representative* of the population. This means that the various groups and types of person in the community are included in the sample to the same extent as they are in the population. You will also have to allow for how *varied* your population is in relation to the information you want (for example, in terms of age, gender, occupation, etc.). If the people are very different, you have to try to ensure that you will include representatives of all the various types by selecting a larger sample or by using some method of selecting from each of the groups (*stratified* sampling). However, the total number of people that you select will be mainly determined by your resources.

If you do not have or cannot compile a list of your population, you can use a *non-probability* sampling method – *quota* sampling, *snowballing* and *purposive* sampling. Here the researcher or the respondent or both influence the selection process. Because this process is not statistically random, it is not possible to assess, with any *confidence* how good a representation your sample is of your population. In exploratory and qualitative studies, this may not be important. However, non-random selection does limit the generalizability of the claims you may make for your results. Non-probability sampling methods are discussed later in this chapter.

Simple random sampling

If you have a suitable population list in which everyone has an equal chance of being selected – one that is not ordered in any way and does not contain duplicates – then you can draw a simple random sample. The most common methods of selection are by lottery, by using random numbers and by systematic sampling. In all of them you will need to know the size of your population and of your sample, and your list must be numbered. This list is referred to as a *sampling frame*.

The *lottery* method is a straightforward and 'fun' method of selection. Here, numbers between one and the number of your total population are written on paper or discs and put into a suitable container. It is important to mix the numbers up in the container to ensure that the last ones in are not on top of the pile. These are then drawn from the container until the sample size is reached. The numbers selected are then checked against the list and the numbered names on the list that correspond to the drawn numbers make up your sample. Clearly, this method is only suitable for small populations.

In larger populations, a method that simulates the draw is the use of *random numbers*. Tables of random numbers are usually included in statistical textbooks or as part of statistical software for computers. If your list is already stored on a computer, you can simply instruct it to select an appropriately sized sample by using its random number routine. Otherwise, you will have to select the numbers manually. Table 5.1 shows an excerpt from a table of random numbers. If you use this method, you will first have to select columns corresponding to the size of your population. Random numbers are then read off down the table until the chosen sample size is obtained. For example, in Table 5.1, we would need to select two of the five columns if our population was two thousand – say we select columns A and B. Starting at any row, we would then read down the rows until our sample size was reached. In this instance, if we started at the first row, the sample would include case 0449 and case 0054, cases 3596, 5980, 4605, 3217 and 6923 would be excluded because they are greater than 2000, then case 1956 would be included etc.

Probably the most common way of selecting a simple random sample is to use a *systematic* method. This can be done by selecting one name from the list, and then counting on another, say, ten places to select the next name, and so on. If we did select every tenth name, we would end up with a sample that was one-tenth the size of the population: a 'one in ten' sample. Although you often hear of them, there is nothing special about one in ten samples. It could be one in three or one in three hundred. The proportion of the population (the *sampling fraction*) you include depends on your resources. For example, in the Winnall study that we discussed in Chapter 2, 274 households were selected using a systematic random sample. This worked out at about one in five households.

A proper systematic random sample should have the first name (or address) selected at random. The easiest way to do this is to add together some numbers like the date, time of day or your age, and use the total you get to count down to the place on the list to find your starting place. Alternatively, you could choose the starting point from a table of random numbers. If your first selection starts by chance in the middle of your list, and counting down comes to the bottom of it, just carry on counting from the top of the list. You have completed your selections when you get back to the name you first started with. This is shown in Figure 5.1.

Table 5.1 *Example of a table of random numbers*

A	B	C	D	E
04	49	35	24	94
00	54	99	76	54
35	96	31	53	07
59	80	80	83	91
46	05	88	52	36
32	17	90	05	97
69	23	46	14	30
19	56	54	14	30
45	15	51	49	38
94	86	43	19	94
75	24	63	38	24
64	05	18	81	59
26	89	80	93	54
45	42	72	68	42
01	39	09	22	86

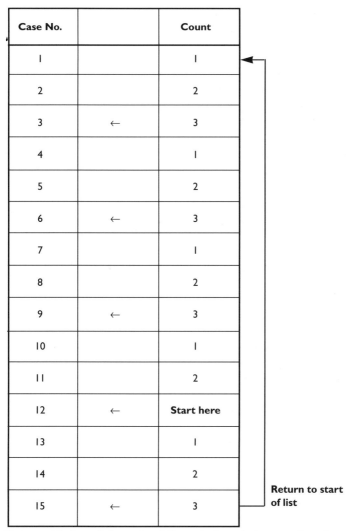

Case No.		Count
1		1
2		2
3	←	3
4		1
5		2
6	←	3
7		1
8		2
9	←	3
10		1
11		2
12	←	Start here
13		1
14		2
15	←	3

Return to start of list

To draw a 1 in 3 sample from a list of 15 people: first calculate a starting point – say, the time of day (18.30 = 12); count the list until you get to the 12th case – this is the first person in your sample; count in threes – every third person will be in your sample until you get to the 12th person again. Those cases with a ← are included in the sample.

Figure 5.1 *Example of a systematic random sample*

Stratified random sampling

In a simple random sample, everyone in your population is treated equally – they all have the same chance of being selected. However, people are not the same. They vary by age, gender, ethnicity, education, employment and many other characteristics, and these might influence their experience, attitudes and health needs. Although adequate for most studies, simple random sampling does not make allowances for this *population variability*. A perfectly sound sample might under-represent certain groups by sheer chance and it will, thus, not be representative of the total population on this characteristic. This is a problem, particularly when the characteristic is rare – those with a particular disease, for example. If you want to make sure that all sections of your population are very accurately represented in the sample in the same proportion as in the population, you can draw a *stratified* sample.

To select a stratified sample, you must first decide which characteristics might influence your study and whether you can identify everyone on your list according to these. For example, you might decide that age was an important distinguishing characteristic. If your list was an electoral roll, you would only be able to divide it into those aged over 17 but under 18 and those over 18. Clearly, this would not be suitable in most cases. However, if you were using a GP's age/sex register, you would be able to group (or 'stratify') your population into whatever age bands you wished. Each group or 'strata' would then become a separate list. You would then be ready to draw a sub-sample from each list using the same sampling fraction (say, one in ten or one in three) by employing any of the simple random sampling methods discussed above. When all lists have been sampled, your overall sample would have the same *proportion* of each group as that of the total population. This is termed *proportional sampling*. For instance, in a study of the health needs of older people, you may decide that those aged 75 years and over are likely to have different needs than the younger group. Your population list consists of 610 people in the 60–74 age group and 390 people in the 75 and over age group (or 61 per cent and 39 per cent, respectively). If you draw a one in five sample from each list, you will obtain 122 from the 60–74 age group and 78 from the 75 and over age group, giving 122/200 (61 per cent) and 78/200 (39 per cent): the same proportions as in your population.

It is also possible to draw a stratified sample *disproportionally*. In populations that include only a small number of people with a particular characteristic, a proportionally drawn sample like the one above might not give enough cases of those with the characteristic from which to derive any meaningful findings. In this case, to achieve an acceptable number of the small group in your sample, a larger number would be selected from this group than from the rest, and the sample would be *disproportional*. For example, in an age stratified sample, you might find that you have 180 people of pensionable age and over and 820 people between 16 and pensionable age. A one in five sample would generate 164 people from the younger age group and only 36 from the older group, which would be far too small for most analytical requirements. Thus, in order to achieve an acceptable number of the older group in your sample, you would change the sampling fraction for this group from one in five to one in three or one in two, say. Here, your overall sample would still contain 164 of the younger group, but the older group would be increased to 60 (one in three) or 90 (one in two). In this case, however, it is important to remember that although the sample is valid, the overall sample is not an accurate representation of your population, and any generalizations that are made from the total sample will be biased towards the over-sampled group.

It is possible to stratify by more than one characteristic. In our examples above, it might be thought necessary to divide the age groups into gender groups, producing four groups rather than two. Obviously, the more strata selected, the more complex your sample design becomes and, for your purposes, it is advisable to limit your design to two strata at the most. Alternatively, you could use a form of *multi-stage* sampling.

Multi-stage sampling

Multi-stage sampling is used when you wish to study people with particular characteristics that are not identifiable on your population list. In this process, each *stage* consists of sampling and screening out until the target group is reached. This group might then all be studied or a final sample drawn from the resulting list. For example, you might want to carry out detailed interviews with mothers of children under 5 who had used a particular brand of baby food. First, you would draw a very large sample from a population list using one of the simple random methods discussed above. This sample would then be surveyed to find out whether they matched the criteria (with children under 5, had used X baby food). From this process, a new population list of those matching the criteria would be drawn up and a sample selected from it. This sample would then be studied in detail.

The main disadvantage of this type of sampling is that it can be fairly expensive and time consuming, and it is probably worth considering other sampling methods if your resources are limited. In the example above, a *cluster* sample of mother and toddler groups or health visitors, for instance, might be suitable. Alternatively, you might use one of the non-probability methods discussed below if you are not overly concerned with the representativeness of your sample.

Cluster sampling

Cluster sampling is used when there is either no readily available population list or when sampling from the whole population would make interviewing too expensive or time consuming. Instead, geographical locations, social groups or time slots are randomly sampled. The population drawn from these *clusters* are then randomly sampled. Either simple or stratified random sampling methods can be used.

Thus, in the example used in multi-stage sampling, instead of listing all women with children under 5 in a city, we might first sample from mother and toddler groups, health visitors or GPs. All women in the selected groups might be interviewed or a further sample could be drawn from the resulting lists.

Quota sampling

Sometimes a random sample is not possible, for example when a list of the population is not available. The main alternative is the *quota sample*. Widely used in market research, this tries to get a sample that is representative by including certain known proportions of the population in the sample. So, for example, we might require that half the sample are men, and half women, because these are the proportions in society at large. We might find from the last Census that locally one in five people are over retirement age, so we could also require that one-fifth of the sample were that age. If unemployment is running at 10 per cent for men and 5 per cent for women, then we might want to ensure our final quota sample has that proportion of those out of paid work. Some examples of this are shown in Figure 5.2. Each person interviewed would then be allocated to one of the selected groups until the categories (quota) had been filled. Interviewers are given a share of each quota to complete.

Although this seems a lot simpler than a random sample – and it is – there are three drawbacks to quota samples. First, to be a reasonably good sample, its quotas have to be treated so that each one connects with the others (as in the above example). So while you may indeed want 80 per cent of people of working age, half of them *also* have to be men *and also*, of these, 10 per cent must not be in paid employment. In the jargon, the quotas *interlock* (see the shaded boxes in Figure 5.2).

When the interviewer starts, she (or he) may pick a woman towards her (or his) quota of female respondents. But that choice will also decide what age and employment quotas are being added to at the same time. In the early stages this is no problem, but as the interviewer nears the end of her selections, the last few combinations become harder to find,

Men				Women		
50				**50**		
Over retirement age	16–retirement age			Over retirement age	16–retirement age	
10	40			10	40	
	Not in paid work	In paid work			Not in paid work	In paid work
	4	36			2	38

The quota of people are then selected to make up the numbers in the shaded boxes.

Figure 5.2 *Example of a quota sample (sample size = 100, over 16 years of age)*

particularly if very detailed breakdowns are devised (for example, occupational groups or narrow age groups). For instance, if the interviewer is left needing to find a man aged over 60 in paid employment, this is a lot harder than finding a younger man in paid work. Depending on the characteristics chosen for the quotas, it may not be possible to fill the interviewer's allocation: a woman aged over 60 and registered as unemployed is a near impossibility. When this happens, the proportions in the sample will not be accurate. Here there is always the risk that interviewers might cheat by fabricating a respondent or by adjusting a respondent's characteristics.

The second problem is who exactly decides who will be interviewed. In random sampling, the interviewer usually has a set of named people to contact. Nobody else can count as valid interviewees. In quota sampling, it is left to the interviewer to decide who gets chosen so long as they meet the quotas. Interviewers can pick people who seem nice or who are easiest to contact, rather than covering the full range of people, and their answers may not be representative. Quota sampling is therefore likely to be less accurate than random sampling.

The third problem is to do with statistics. For mathematical reasons, some statistical techniques only work reliably when the data come from random samples. This is particularly significant in measuring the accuracy of the estimates that the sample gives you of what the population's answers would be. It is not possible to know how good your estimates will be with a quota sample.

Because of these limitations, research based on quota samples tends to be treated as less reliable. If you are seeking to convince bureaucrats, politicians and health professionals, your case will be more credible if you have been able to use a random sample. On the other hand, constraints of time, volunteers, or budgets may leave you no option. While random sampling is better, quota sampling, if carefully done, is a good second choice.

Snowballing

A *snowballing* or *pyramid* sampling method can be used when no population list is available and representativeness is not regarded as important for the investigation. Here, researchers first select people known to them who are appropriate to the study. These people are interviewed and asked to nominate people known to them who fit the selection criteria. These are then interviewed, and so on, until a suitably sized sample is obtained. Thus, in the women with children under 5 example, you would first approach women known to you (or if you knew none, known to some of your friends or colleagues). You would then interview these women and ask them to name other women with children under 5, etc., at each stage making sure that you did not approach previous respondents.

This is a very simple and cheap method of obtaining detailed information from people who are not easily identified. However, the resulting sample is likely to be extremely biased towards the particular social groups that you or your first set of respondents belong to. Your findings will, therefore, be of limited generalizability.

Purposive sampling

In this method of selection, researchers *purposely* select people whom they think might contribute useful information. These people are often referred to as *key informants* or *expert witnesses*. Here, particular groups of people, such as teachers, police, GPs, councillors, chairpersons of community organizations, shopkeepers etc. are selected. The main disadvantage of this method is that, although it is relatively quick, the views of these people are not necessarily representative of the whole community. *Rapid Appraisal*, discussed in Chapter 8, relies heavily on this type of sample. Purposive sampling is most useful in the early stages of a project, to get an idea of the range of issues that might be important to include in a questionnaire, or as part of a multi-method study, but it is very limited as the main method of assessing needs.

There are many examples of this type of sampling. In a study carried out in a local authority housing estate in Edinburgh, the research team interviewed community workers and professionals (teachers, health visitors, etc.), community leaders and 17 residents who were selected to represent various age groups, social situations and health problems (Murray and Graham, 1995). This sample formed only part of the study, which also included a survey of a GP practice's patients and the use of existing information.

Volunteers

Using volunteers is becoming an increasingly popular method of selecting respondents by non-professionals, for example in magazine surveys. Although it seems a fairly straightforward and obvious way of getting respondents, it should be avoided if at all possible. Using volunteers might be seen as the opposite of purposive sampling. By volunteering, people *choose* to be among those selected. This recruitment might be through public meetings, advertisements or by word of mouth. These methods of selection have the same limitations as purposive sampling since volunteers are unlikely to be representative of the whole community. Further, whereas in purposive selection by researcher you are likely to know why you chose particular respondents, with volunteers you do not know why they have volunteered. Again, as with purposive selection, the use of volunteers is useful for preliminary or exploratory research, or in a mixed-methods approach. However, it should not be used as the only method of collecting information.

Bowling's (1993) study in City and Hackney used a version of this type of sampling in the community group phase of the project. Here, questionnaires were distributed to those attending meetings of various community organizations. In contrast, Gordon (1992) used a radio broadcast to recruit subjects for her study of women suffering from depression. Volunteers were then screened for eligibility.

Sample size

Some textbooks deal at length with methods of calculating the correct sample size. This is relevant for large scale, well funded research where precise estimates are essential, and various statistical formulae and look-up tables have been produced to determine correct sample sizes (see, for example, Sarantakos, 1993: 144–50). However, these are largely irrelevant for your purposes, and the size will be determined by your resources and the type of investigation you are carrying out. In general, the variability of your population will determine the sample size – if it is large, the sample should be large – since you should aim for a sample

Table 5.2 *Population list for the sampling exercise*

No.	Age	Gender	No.	Age	Gender
1	A	M	26	A	M
2	A	M	27	A	F
3	A	F	28	A	F
4	A	F	29	A	F
5	A	F	30	A	M
6	B	F	31	A	F
7	B	M	32	A	M
8	A	F	33	B	M
9	A	F	34	A	F
10	A	M	35	B	M
11	A	F	36	A	F
12	A	F	37	A	F
13	A	F	38	A	M
14	B	M	39	A	M
15	A	F	40	A	M
16	A	M	41	A	F
17	A	M	42	A	F
18	A	M	43	B	M
19	B	F	44	B	F
20	A	M	45	A	F
21	A	M	46	A	F
22	B	F	47	A	M
23	A	F	48	B	F
24	A	F	49	A	F
25	A	F	50	A	F

Age: A = 64 and under; B = 65 and over.

that is as representative as possible of your population. In qualitative studies, where representativeness is not usually as important as the richness of the data, smaller samples with more detailed information from each respondent is acceptable. A good idea of the sample size you should aim for can be obtained by looking at existing reports that are concerned with similar investigations.

Chapter summary

This chapter has reviewed the main methods of selecting respondents. Rather than seeking information from everyone in a chosen *population*, it is usual to select a small number who are *representative* of the whole.

If you have a list of your population (a *sampling frame*), you can use any one of a range of *random* methods to draw a *sample*. These include *simple, stratified, multi-stage* and *cluster* sampling. The main advantage of random methods is that you can calculate how good an estimate your sample is of the population from which it was drawn, and therefore how close your sample findings are to those obtained if you had collected information from the whole group.

When there is no suitable sampling frame, or if you are not too concerned with generalizability, you can use a *non-random selection* technique. The main ones are *quota* and *purposive* sampling, *snowballing* and using *volunteers*. These last three methods should not be used if you want to make general statements or do any statistical analysis.

Exercise

In Table 5.2, a population of fifty is listed with details of age and gender.

1 Draw a one in five simple random sample from the table.
2 Draw a one in five random sample stratified by gender from the table.
3 List ten people that you know, giving details of their age and gender.
4 In Table 5.2, 40 per cent of the population are males and 60 per cent are females. Of these, 80 per cent are 64 years of age and under, and 20 per cent are 65 years of age and over. How do the three samples you have drawn compare with these?

CHAPTER 6

ASKING QUESTIONS

Asking questions of other people (*respondents*) is the principal way of obtaining information in social research. For even when methods such as observation are used it is usual to ask some questions. However, although it may seem like everyday conversation, questioning for research is different. In the research setting, questions are determined by the aims and objectives of the study. Their construction may involve highly structured techniques and, in all cases, the recording of the answers is extremely important.

This chapter discusses the methods of deciding what questions to ask and how to ask them. Whether you are conducting quantitative or qualitative research you will first need to draw up a *topic list* and, if you intend to undertake a social survey, you will have to design a *questionnaire*. In quantitative research you have to decide whether to use *self-completion* or *survey interviewing* to obtain your information. Qualitative studies involve interviewing techniques that are far less structured than those used in surveys. Here, where detail and richness are of primary importance, *depth interviewing*, *group discussions* and self-completion techniques such as *diaries* are employed.

Topic lists

The first stage in determining what questions you need to ask is to write down a list of topics that you want to cover. This is usually obtained from preliminary discussions and looking at similar studies that have already been carried out. For example, the study of local needs undertaken in Leeds (Percy-Smith and Sanderson, 1992) used Doyal and Gough's list of 'intermediate needs' as a basis for their study (see Chapter 1, above). This list, and those used in other studies referred to in this book, are listed in Table 6.1. Once you have drawn up a list, each topic is translated into one or more questions.

Table 6.1. *Topics used in health and community research*

1 From Percy-Smith and Sanderson (1992)
General health
Psychological health
Social and leisure activities
Education
Diet
Housing
Employment and work conditions
Environment
Health services
Social services
Family and friends
Income and wealth
Crime
Autonomy and control over life
Children and future

2 From Burton (1993)
Demographic (age, gender, etc.)
Housing
Economic
Environment
Health and welfare
Local services

3 From Compass Handbook (1996)
Housing
Crime
Employment
Income
Education and training
Environment
Health and welfare

4 Rapid Appraisal topics

Health policy	National and local government policies.
Education services	Schools, colleges, nurseries etc.
Health services	GPs, community nurses, clinics, hospitals, chemists, dentists etc.
Social services	Social, probation and community development workers, public housing, benefits etc.
Physical environment	Buildings, land, roads, transport, pollution etc.
Socio-economic environment	Jobs, income, families, leisure facilities, clubs and organizations etc.
Disease and disability	Physical and mental illness, impairment, deaths.

5 Medical categories
(see Glossary for definitions)
Birth rate
Infant mortality rates (IMRs)
Low birthweight rates
Standard mortality ratios (SMRs)
Morbidity rates
Department of Health targets
Immunization rates

Designing a questionnaire

The questions that are asked in survey research are usually highly standardized so that everyone in the sample is asked the same questions,
in the same order. This means that all the questions have to be written
down in a standardized form (*questionnaire*) even if they are going to be
asked by an interviewer. Designing a questionnaire is a specialist skill
and, if you have never done this before, you should seriously consider
seeking help from someone with expert knowledge. Alternatively, you
might consider using questions from existing studies or packages (these
are discussed in Chapter 8, below). There are also specialist texts on
questionnaire design that you might refer to: for example, Oppenheim,
(1992). However, whatever method you use, you will still need to draw
up a list of topics that you would like to be included. Your list then has
to be converted into easily understandable and answerable questions.
These should be designed not to offend and not to take up too much
time.

The wording and order of the questions will be influenced by the
way in which you are going to collect the information: by a self-
completion questionnaire or by an interviewer. An interviewer can use
prompts, probes and show cards, and will ask the questions in the order
they appear. If you want the respondents to complete the questionnaire
themselves, you must take into account that they might not answer the
questions in the same order and they could ask the opinion of others in
their household.

In designing the questionnaire, there are certain basic rules that
should always be followed. These can be divided into pitfalls (what you
should avoid), types of questions, and question order.

Pitfalls

In our professional lives we all tend to use specialist jargon, and sometimes this spills over into our everyday speech. Some of our contacts
will understand the terms we use, others will ask what we mean or
poke fun at us, and still others will pretend to know and/or misinter-
pret what we say. In designing a questionnaire it is important to make
the questions easily understandable to all of your respondents. Each
question should mean the same to everyone involved so that comparable answers are obtained. Thus the language used should be *simple,
non-technical* and *unambiguous*. For example, a survey relating to eating
patterns should not include questions about 'adequate nutritional
requirements' or even 'a balanced diet', since many people would either
not understand the terms used or not know what constituted

'adequate', 'nutritional', 'balanced' or 'diet'. Instead, respondents might be asked what they ate and drank during a particular day or their last meal. Here, note that 'ate and drank' is used rather than 'consumed': always use the simplest vocabulary you can. Designing questionnaires is difficult. You know what you mean, but do others have a similar understanding of the question? This might be minimized if you always try to draft with another person. Then try it out on your family and friends to see if it works.

Questions that appear to expect a certain answer (*leading* questions) should not be used in a questionnaire. This is because respondents are likely to agree with the sentiments expressed in the question because they think it is the correct answer, rather than giving their own opinion. For example, 'Youth crime is a problem in this area, isn't it?' would be better phrased as 'Do you think that youth crime is a problem in this area?' or, even better, 'Which of the following do you think is the main problem in this area?', followed by a list of possible problems.

Questions that combine two or more questions into one should also be avoided, but they are still very commonly included in many surveys. These are the *that and that* questions. For instance, 'Do you think that this area should have more recreational facilities and day care centres for children and older people?' Here, you will not know whether the answer is to 'recreational centres' or 'day care centres' for 'children' or 'older people'. The question should become two or, perhaps, even four separate questions.

Another form of question to be avoided is that illustrated by the old chestnut 'When did you stop beating your wife?' Such *threatening* questions or those that might arouse *anxiety* are best substituted by more general questions or a different type of study. For example, a study of child abuse might include questions listing a range of physical and mental abuses to ascertain those that a respondent thought most serious. Alternatively, a different type of study could be considered. Although this example is about criminal activity, it is important to be aware that people feel threatened or anxious about a range of topics.

Questions that involve *mental arithmetic* or that need *detailed memory recall* may also cause anxiety. Further, they are likely to obtain a high proportion of factually incorrect answers. Thus, a question asking for the average age of the people living in a household would require the respondent not only to know the ages of everyone but also know how to calculate averages. Instead, it is preferable to ask for the individual ages and calculate the averages afterwards or at the data analysis stage.

A final pitfall in questionnaire design is the inclusion of questions that are far *too general*. For example, 'What do you think about this area?' might obtain a wider range of non-comparable answers such as 'not a lot' or a very detailed account of the history, environment and social life of the area. Alternatives to such questions include using a list of statements that the respondent can agree or disagree with, or you might ask about specific features of the area separately. General questions do, however, have a role to play as introductory questions. These are principally included to put the respondent at ease rather than to provide any data.

Types of questions

There are two main types of questions used in questionnaires: *open-ended* and *closed*. Open-ended questions are those that leave the answer entirely to the respondent. For example, 'What do you think are the main health problems in this area?' Such questions are included when there is little prior knowledge of the range of possible responses or when the researcher feels that more detailed responses might add more depth to the survey, or as opening/closing questions.

Closed questions, on the other hand, usually form the majority of questions. These give a fixed number of answers from which a respondent may choose one or more. Here the researcher has enough previous knowledge of the possible responses before undertaking the study. However, often categories such as 'Other' or 'Don't Know' are included to allow for wider variations. The main advantage of these questions is that they are easily classified at the coding stage, or can often be pre-coded on the questionnaire. In this case, each possible answer is given a code value that is printed adjacent to the particular response. Coding is discussed in Chapter 9.

Closed questions can take a number of forms. The most common of which are *check list* questions. These offer a number of alternatives. For example, 'How do you travel to work?: walk; cycle; car; bus; train; mixture of these; other'. Here, only one answer can be selected. Alternatively, the respondent may be allowed to select a fixed number of answers or as many as necessary: 'Which of the following foods have you eaten today?: bread; rice; pasta; potatoes; pastry; eggs; meat; lentils; beans; fruit; green vegetables'.

Ratings and *rankings* are types of closed questions that measure people's attitudes or opinions. The range of replies to these is in the form of some type of scaling method, ranging from 'strongly agree' to 'strongly disagree'. These are usually referred to as 'Likert-type' scale questions after one of the most famous scales. For example, 'Most people today are concerned about their health. Do you strongly agree/agree/ neither agree nor disagree/ disagree/strongly disagree'. Alternatively, a hypothetical range of values is given in which one end of the scale is one extreme and the other end is the opposite extreme. For instance, 'How would you rate your health on the following scale?

Very good (1) —––––— Very poor (10)'. A thorough account of these scaling techniques is given in Oppenheim (1992).

Often respondents are only required to answer certain questions if they have answered a previous question in a particular way. This question is called a *contingency* or *filter* question. Clearly, to work, filter questions have to be closed. For example, you may only want to ask questions about children's ailments of those respondents with children under 10 years of age. Here, you would first of all ask if they had children under 10 years old – the *filter* – and then direct the flow of questions to those concerning children's ailments using, for example, 'If Yes, go to Question 9'. These instructions also give rise to the term 'skip' or 'GOTO' questions.

In surveys that use interviewers to collect information, it is possible to print the responses to closed questions on *show cards*. Here, each response is given a letter or digit and respondents are asked to select their response to a particular question from this list. This can save time when a number of questions have the same range of possible responses, when the list is very long or when sensitive questions are being asked, because the interviewer only has to read out the question and not the list. For example, it is more likely that a truthful response to a question on, say, cigarette smoking will be given if the respondent can read off 'H' from a card rather than saying 'over 40 a day' to the interviewer.

With an interview survey it is also possible to obtain more information by using *prompts* and *probes*. Prompts and probes are methods used to encourage a respondent to give more information (prompts) or to expand on what has already been said (probes). Prompts include phrases such as 'Is there anything else that *you think is a main health problem in this area ?'* (here part of the question is repeated); or '*Are there any other leisure activities that you do? (repeat list)'*. Here, 'Anything else?' or 'Any other?' are used until the interviewer is satisfied that a complete answer has been obtained in a multiple choice or open-ended question. Probes include such phrases as 'What do you mean by . . . (repeat what the respondent has said)?'. Here the interviewer attempts to clarify a statement made by the respondent. Note that in such instances the questions or answers are repeated in full or in part. Paraphrasing is not allowed because of the danger of interviewers biasing the response.

Question order

The order in which you ask questions has an important influence on the answers. It is not usual to ask personal questions (about income etc.) at the beginning because you might get a hostile response and a refusal to continue. Generally, questions are designed to flow into each other so that the rules of a normal conversation are followed. Sometimes, however, it is possible to hide a question amongst other topics as a way of checking previous responses. Questions can also be in a narrowing or broadening sequence. In a narrowing or 'funnelling' sequence, general questions are asked first, followed by increasingly specific ones. A broadening sequence is one where specific questions are asked, followed by increasingly general ones. However, it must be noted that in self-completion questionnaires no order can be assumed because respondents can choose their own order.

Piloting

After you have constructed your draft questionnaire, it is usual to pilot (or trial) it. No one – not even experts – gets the questions right first time and preliminary testing is vital. Piloting is a way of testing not only the question wording, order, range of responses and instructions, but also the introductory explanation or covering letter and the overall length. Usually piloting is done by first trying out the questionnaire on members of your group, family, neighbours and friends. After these initial tests, and further design refinements, a small sample of actual respondents is used for a wider pilot. The interviewers and others involved in the exercise then meet to discuss possible problems and changes before the final version of the questionnaire is designed. The questions that you need to ask of those involved in the piloting are:

- Did people understand what the survey was about and why you were doing it?
- Were any questions difficult to ask/read?
- Were any questions difficult to answer?
- Were the answers to the questions what you expected?
- Were the questions misinterpreted?
- Did the range of choices cover the majority of responses or was there a high proportion of 'other' responses?
- Did any of the questions appear irrelevant (high proportion of non-response, don't know answers)?
- Did the filter questions work?
- Did the show cards work?
- How long did the questionnaire take to complete?

At this stage it is also possible to decide on a coding scheme for processing the information. Coding schemes are discussed in Chapter 9.

Administering surveys

You will need to have decided on a method of collecting the information before you design your questionnaire. Basically there are two ways to do this: interviewing respondents or asking them to write down the answers themselves. In both cases it is important to inform the police, and interviewers should be issued with identity cards.

Interviewing

Survey interviews are carried out either *face-to-face* with the respondent or by phone. In needs assessment surveys these will usually be carried out face-to-face. This type of interview has the advantage of establishing a closer relationship with the respondents and is thus less likely to be refused than other methods. A further advantage of interviewing over self-completion is that more useful information can be obtained from any open-ended questions that you have included: an interviewer can prompt by asking 'Anything else?'.

Although interviewers might approach people in the street (in quota sampling for example, see Chapter 5 above), in this type of study it is more likely that they will approach people in their own homes. These interviews can be pre-arranged (by letter or phone) or the interviewer can call at a random time. Usually in interview surveys each respondent is given a letter explaining the nature and purpose of the interview, and the interviewer will be given a standard introductory statement to say. Interviewers will be instructed on how to handle any problems that might arise and should always be polite and not demanding.

No survey has a 100 per cent response rate (even the Census does not achieve this!). The reasons for this are because of people not being in, people moving or dying, or the address or person is unknown. Standardized procedures have been developed to tackle these problems. If people have died, moved out of the area, cannot be traced, or if the address or person is unknown, a replacement is made. (It is usual to draw up a list of substitutes/reserves when you select your sample.) These are not counted as non-response. In the case of people not being in, the interviewer is instructed to call back twice more, at different times of the day, before a non-contact is recorded.

Only a very few people will refuse to be interviewed if the survey is being carried out correctly. In this case interviewers should attempt to find out the reason for the refusal. It might be because they called at an inconvenient time, in which case a more suitable time could be arranged. Other reasons include fear, worry about their views becoming known, or that they feel that they do not know anything about the topic. The interviewer should attempt to reassure them about these issues. Figure 6.1 shows these different categories of response and the actions to be taken.

Self-completion questionnaires

These surveys are much quicker and cheaper to undertake than interviews, although you will have to provide reply-paid envelopes or arrange for them to be collected. Again, as with interviewer call-backs, it is usual to send out at least one reminder. However, except for specialist-type surveys, they have much lower response rates, and thus the cost per response is higher. Because you are relying on people filling in the forms themselves, you will have to be even more careful with the instructions, the wording of the questions and the range of topics and types of questions you include. Also, some people may not be able to complete a questionnaire because they are visually or physically disabled or they have problems understanding the questions because of language or comprehension difficulties.

After three reminders the response rate to the postal questionnaire used in the City and Hackney study (Bowling, 1993) was only 10 per cent gross (45 out of 454) or 11 per cent net (when movers etc. were

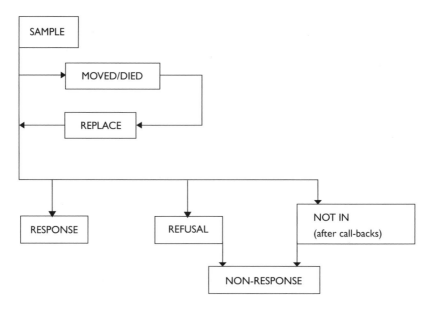

Figure 6.1 *Respondent outcomes*

discounted). It was therefore decided to interview the remainder. Of the 353 people remaining, 265 responded to the interview survey. This gave an overall net response rate of 77 per cent (310 out of 398). In discussing this Bowling concludes:

> One lesson to be learnt from this study . . . is that a postal survey is *not* the method of choice when aiming to target a random sample of the public: response is likely to be poor. Moreover, this exercise showed that members of Black populations were less likely to respond to the postal questionnaire than to the interview. (Bowling, 1993: 59)

Because of such difficulties, self-completion surveys are probably best restricted to interest-based groups or form part of a larger study. For example, the postal questionnaire survey of medical practitioners in Bowling's study achieved a 67 per cent response rate.

It is generally thought that a high *response rate* is a good thing. This is not always the case. As discussed in Chapter 5, the main aim of a sample is to be *a good representation* of the population from which it was selected. Thus, a response rate of 10 per cent may be adequate if it contains different groups in the same proportion as they are distributed in the population. On the other hand, a response rate of 80 per cent may not be a good representation if the remaining 20 per cent are all from one particular group.

In order to find out how representative your respondents are of the total population, it is usual to produce a comparative table. This would compare the known characteristics of the population as shown in the Census with those of your respondents. The example shown in Table 6.2 is a shortened version of one produced for the City and Hackney study (Bowling, 1993). This shows a clear *under-representation* of the under-30 age group and an *over-representation* of the 30–60 age group.

Explanations and instructions

As well as producing a questionnaire, you will need to provide a brief explanation of the survey and instructions about filling it in. The format of these will depend on how you are going to collect the information: by using interviewers or by self-completion.

If you use interviewers, you will need to decide on what they will say to respondents as an introduction to themselves and the survey. In surveys it is important that each interviewer uses the same wording – you 'write their script'. Some interview surveys also provide a short letter of explanation that is given to each respondent. If you are using a self-completion questionnaire, the explanation will be in the form of a covering letter.

Table 6.2 *Characteristics of Bowling's random sample of the public in comparison with 1991 Census data for Hackney*

	Responders (%)	% total population, Hackney 1991 Census estimate
Gender		
Female	56	51
Male	44	49
Ethnic group		
White UK/European	50	52
Black	50	48
Age		
<30	30	48
30>60	58	36
60+	12	16

Source: adapted from Bowling, 1993: 33

Whatever method you use, your explanation should include the following information:

- Who you/your group are.
- A *brief description* of the survey, *why* you are doing it and *what* you hope to *achieve* (for example, more play areas, a health centre, to argue a case for more money to be invested in your community etc.).
- How the person being interviewed has been selected.
- The confidentiality of the information.
- Stress the need for *their* views, opinion, etc.
- The name, address and telephone number of someone they can contact about the survey/interviewer's credentials.
- Thank them for their cooperation.

Remember that respondents are *doing you a favour* by giving you their time and information, so that interviewers should be polite and persuasive rather than pushy and aggressive.

A self-completion questionnaire will have to have very clear instructions about filling it in and *who* should fill it in. You should make it clear *how* you want people to indicate their answers – tick, cross, circle or by deleting the answers that do not apply. Also, make it clear how many answers they can give to a question: for example, 'TICK ALL THAT APPLY', 'TICK ONE BOX ONLY'. Filter questions and those that you want only certain people to answer should also be clearly labelled. You might also use a different size or style of lettering to distinguish questions from instructions. An example of a letter giving an explanation of a survey and instructions for completing the questionnaire is given in Figure 6.2.

The layout of a questionnaire should be neat and clear — 'easy on the eye' – and it should always be typed. The type size should be large enough to read easily so that it does not appear cramped or look 'cheap'. Sufficient space should also be allowed for a complete answer. People have different-sized handwriting and this should always be taken into consideration. Because computer software packages now make it easy to use different fonts for the text and include various other graphic elements (clip art, for example), there is a temptation to include too many elements. The overall effect is often too 'busy'. Remember that the main aim is to design a questionnaire that is easy to read and complete rather than to create an art object or to demonstrate your new software.

Response record/summary sheets

Whatever type of sample you take, it is important to keep a record of completed interviews/returned questionnaires and issues raised by

---

Dear Patient

SURVEY ON AMBULANCE/PATIENT TRANSPORT SERVICES IN THE PLYMOUTH AREA. YOUR JOURNEY TO & FROM HOSPITAL OR CLINIC TODAY

The Community Health Council (CHC) is looking at the Quality of AMBULANCE/PATIENT TRANSPORT SERVICES in the PLYMOUTH area, we are asking you to help by completing the questionnaire and posting it back to us in the envelope provided. This form and your opinions are confidential and you do not need to give your name and address.

Please use a blue or black pen and mark the relevant box with a cross as shown here ☒. On most questions you should only put a cross in one box. Please print where comment is asked for, and if there are any remarks you wish to make about any question, please use the space under each question.

The CHC has a statutory duty to monitor aspects of the National Health Service and to recommend improvements. On occasions we do this by conducting surveys of patients views.

In the new year the results of the survey will be available. If you would like to receive this information please get in touch with this office.

I would like to thank you, in advance, for helping the Council with the survey.
Yours sincerely,

Figure 6.2 *Example of a cover letter* (Plymouth Community Health Council, n.d.)

interviewers. This will enable you to monitor progress and to decide whether you need to draw a further sample and make replacements. For interview surveys it is essential to keep a record of each interviewer's quota/contact list and progress.

The selection and training of survey interviewers

Interviewers, or potential interviewers, have to have good interpersonal skills; average intelligence, the ability to work on their own, be trustworthy, have a knowledge of the locality and, of special importance in community studies, not be identified as belonging to any particular interest group or clique within the community. Beyond these basic guidelines, it is probably best to select interviewers by observing their performance during the training period.

Training interviewers involves both general training in interviewing techniques and specific briefing about the particular survey that they will be doing. Perhaps the best way of doing this is through a series of workshops, with broad topics discussed with the whole group and more detailed training in small groups and trial sessions. The following points should be covered:

- General principles of surveys (samples, types of questions).
- Confidentiality.
- Truthfulness.
- Presentation of self and personal appearance – tidy but not too smart.
- How to gain cooperation and trust.
- The importance of reading the questions exactly as they are worded.
- Prompting and probing techniques.
- Accuracy in recording answers.
- Personal protection and safety.
- Essential items to carry: identity card, covering letters, telephone numbers, addresses of respondents, folder, blank questionnaires, maps, pens and pencils, show cards.
- Issues relating to the particular survey: preferably a handbook should be prepared. Interviewers should be taken through the questionnaire and also have time to conduct some trial interviews.

In addition to briefing interviewers before the survey is undertaken, it is important to *debrief* them when it is completed (and during the study, if it continues for a long period). Here, not only should the issues raised in the pilot stage be covered, but also the overall perceptions of the interviewers: how the interviews went, difficult questions, difficult groups, any information that was not included in the questionnaire.

The following example summarizes the conclusions from the debriefing session in the Winnall project.

> The interviewers encountered less non-cooperation than anticipated. They also found residents helpful and pleased that something was being done for Winnall. Residents appeared grateful that the interviewers did not represent local statutory authorities. The surveys themselves were rather long although the content did appear to cover the main areas of residents' concerns. The best survey techniques tended to be operating in pairs with one interviewer asking questions and the second interviewer writing down the responses. This technique was not used all the time, but on evaluation was suggested the best option. Those interviewers that were residents themselves felt that they were better able to empathise with the concerns raised during the survey and believed their local knowledge was a positive factor during the interviews. (Winnall Neighbourhood Forum, 1993: 14)

Depth interviewing

Unlike the survey interview, depth interviewing relies on the interpersonal skills and knowledge of the interviewer as an initiator of topics rather than on a carefully worded questionnaire. However, interviewers have to be careful to avoid expressing their own opinions or suggesting answers. As the name suggests, the aim of this type of interview is to obtain an in-depth account of particular topics.

Potential respondents may be selected by one of the sampling techniques discussed in Chapter 5 or they may be volunteers. Qualitative methods are less concerned with representativeness and generalizability than with the variety and depth of feelings, meanings and understandings etc. Usually, these interviews are conducted in the respondents' homes and, because they can take a long time, are prearranged. Respondents are normally informed about the nature and broad subject matter of the interview beforehand and are therefore likely to have thought about their views, and possibly discussed these with others.

As part of the study that explored the health needs of black and ethnic minority women in Glasgow, the Community Support Group carried out depth interviews with key workers. These included community workers, race relations officers, medical practitioners and nurses. Rather than selecting this group by random sampling techniques, they were chosen 'so as to ensure a diversity of ideas, experience, knowledge and perspectives' (Avan, 1995: 6). Other examples of depth interviewing include the Dumbiedykes study (Murray and Graham, 1995) and the *Rapid Appraisal* studies reported by Ong and Humphris (1994).

Semi-structured (or 'focused') interviews are based on a small number of open-ended questions, the answers to which are *probed* (see above) by the interviewer for clarification or elaboration. Often a subset of topics are listed, so that the interviewer might concentrate on these issues. The questions or topics have to be put in the order that they appear on the question sheet (*interview schedule*). The respondent can then be led from a general first question to more specific ones.

The *unstructured* (or non-directive) interview is the least structured form of interview. No pre-defined questions are given and there is no ordering of topics. Instead, topics are often simply listed as an *aide-mémoire*. Here, the aim of the interview is for respondents to give their accounts of their experiences, opinions and feelings on particular issues in their own way. The interviewer's task is to probe for further details and ask for clarification when necessary. Thus, the questions the interviewer might ask would be determined by the particular interview. These questions should not, however, express the interviewer's own opinions or bias the respondent's account. Usually interviewers are given general guidelines, but no written instructions are used. This type of interview often requires interviewers to have detailed knowledge of the issues so that suitable probing and supplementary questions can be asked.

Obviously these interviews cannot be recorded on a standard form, and copious note taking might inhibit the flow of the interview. Instead, tape or video recorders are normally used if the respondent is agreeable. These should be placed as unobtrusively as possible and the interviewer should change tapes in a way that avoids too much interruption to the flow of the interview. Some notes should be made if at all possible in case of mechanical failure. The recording should be checked for any problems as soon as possible afterwards.

Things can go wrong, however well prepared, and a good memory is an asset. For example, after completing an unstructured interview for a study of childless couples (Payne, 1978), I returned to my car and checked my recording to find that the tape had snarled up. I drove around the corner and wrote down as much of the interview as possible. As it happened, by good fortune, I was later able to rescue most of the tape. My hastily written notes had given a fairly accurate account of the recording. Had I waited for the tape to be transcribed, I would probably have forgotten much of the detail of the interview.

The transcription of recordings is probably the most tedious and time consuming aspect of these interviewing methods. It is usual for the recordings to be transcribed verbatim into readable text. This can then be manually processed or input into a text-coding computer program (see Chapter 10). In the Glasgow study mentioned above, the report stresses the importance of recording *everything* that is said so that a complete picture can be obtained.

Group discussions

In our everyday lives, our ideas, opinions, feelings and attitudes are formed or influenced by our contacts with others. Unlike the methods previously discussed, the use of group discussions attempts to reflect this by obtaining information from people in groups. These can range from large public meetings and forums to highly specialized *focus groups* involving about eight to ten people.

Because of group dynamics, it is unlikely that everyone will speak at a large meeting. The views expressed are therefore unlikely to be representative: the opinions will be those of community leaders, 'experts' and those who regularly attend meetings. This form of group discussion is a collective version of conducting individual interviews with key informants. They are useful in the early stages of a project, as a means of getting a feel of the issues and topics to explore. However, if used as a main method of investigation, they are likely to reflect the opinions of the vocally or politically dominant members rather than the whole range of community views.

It might be argued that those who work with or represent the community are likely to have a good idea of what 'the community at large' may feel on particular issues. This is not necessarily the case. Views raised and expressed to these people are likely to be influenced by their particular function in the community. Further, these community representatives usually only meet a sub-section of the population. GPs, local councillors and MPs, for example, only have knowledge of patients or constituents who consult them.

In order to overcome these problems, a series of smaller discussion groups or *focus groups* could be held. Focus groups are a special type of group discussion, first used by Robert Merton, an American sociologist, in 1956 (Merton et al., 1956). The techniques for conducting them have since been carefully developed by market research companies, although they are now being widely used in the public sector. Recently they have become a topic of media attention because of their use by political parties as a method of assessing public opinion. It is becoming increasingly common to find any form of group discussion incorrectly described as a focus group. Focus groups are far more formal than other forms of group discussion. Here, members should not know each other and should preferably be similar to each other in terms of education, social status, occupation and income etc.

As implied by the name, focus groups *focus* on particular issues that are introduced in a predetermined order as carefully worded open-ended questions or topics. Those invited to attend might be from various sections of the community, or a series of discussions could be held with particular interest groups (for example, community leaders, teenagers, women, the elderly). This approach was used in the Glasgow study of the health needs of black and ethnic minority women (Avan, 1995) and the health priorities research in City and Hackney (Bowling, 1993).

In each of these examples existing groups were approached and discussions were held with those groups that agreed to participate. Bowling found that on the one occasion that a 'mixed' group was used very little useful information was obtained. As an alternative to using existing groups sampling procedures could be used. For example, a study carried out for Somerset Health Authority used sampling procedures to select focus group membership (Richardson and Bowie, 1995). This would help to ensure that the full range of community opinion was represented rather than groups being dominated by 'professional volunteers'. These groups should normally consist of between six and ten people, and any more than twelve has been found to inhibit the discussion.

When organizing such discussions, it is important to arrange a suitable location (one that is accessible for all attendees and is comfortable) and a convenient time. In addition, it is important to remember that people may have problems attending meetings because of family or employment commitments. To ensure a good attendance, financial inducements or small gifts are sometimes given to those attending (the Somerset study paid each person £10). Additionally, transport and crèche facilities may be provided, and it is usual to supply some form of refreshment: tea, coffee etc.

Focus groups are extremely useful for finding out about underlying issues and opinions and for discovering how views and attitudes are formed. Comments and opinions made by members can trigger a whole range of views from others in the group. These groups can be non-directive around a general topic (similar to the unstructured one-to-one interview) or concentrated on particular questions (like the semi-structured interview). They are widely used in consultative health projects and community profiling as an aid to planning and prioritizing, for the evaluation of programmes and in needs assessment. For example, the Person-to-Person project in Bristol used focus groups as their principal method of consultation in response to *Local Voices* (NHS Management Executive, 1992) and Somerset Health Authority used them to assist in their resource allocation decisions (Richardson and Bowie, 1995; Shepherd, 1995).

The *Priority Search* approach, discussed in Chapter 8, is based on a general question that has previously been decided (for example, 'What would improve your health, happiness and well-being?' (Priority Search, 1994)). Other examples use a small number of previously selected topics on which to concentrate the discussion. Those attending group discussions in the City and Hackney study were first asked to complete a questionnaire. This was then used as a basis for the discussions that followed. In the programme undertaken for Somerset Health Authority, attendees were given briefing notes and a list of topics beforehand and an expert was on hand to deal with specialist queries (Richardson and Bowie, 1995).

The interviewer, now often called the *facilitator*, has to use different skills and techniques than in the one-to-one interview. The interviewer is given a very detailed briefing and often, as in the Somerset study discussed above, an expert is on hand to give additional information. The methods of question construction and interviewer probing and control are the same as those previously discussed, but with the added problems of group control. Here, the interviewer must control the discussion so that only one person speaks at a time, everyone is encouraged to speak in turn and no one dominates. In this last case, the interviewer needs to be able to say 'shut up' without sounding threatening or inhibiting the others. Seating arrangements can also be used to influence participation. The more reticent members should be seated opposite the facilitator so that eye contact can be used to encourage them to join in. In contrast, the vociferous should be seated in a position that makes it difficult for them to catch the eye of the facilitator.

It is also common to use a second interviewer (or *scribe*) to operate the tape recorder and act as note-taker, and usually name badges or place names are used to aid the transcription process. As a general rule, interviewers should not be members of the community or at least not be identified with any particular faction, and not be known to members of the group. The location of the meeting is also important. It should be accessible, comfortable and non-threatening, so that people will feel free to talk and share their experiences and opinions.

Focus groups – a warning

Because of their recent high media profile, by being used by the British Labour Party under Tony Blair and the Clinton administration in the US, there is a tendency for focus groups to be used indiscriminately and inappropriately. The term is increasingly used, particularly in community-based research, to describe group discussions that are little more than 'chats' or substitutes for action. The dangers here are obvious. Unless correctly understood, managed and prepared, information derived from them can have little validity or usefulness. Focus groups are best employed when research is needed to find out about underlying issues and opinions, and the *process* of attitude formation. They are not a substitute for a community survey. When there is a lack of understanding about the limitations of the method, there is a great danger that unsubstantiated generalizations might be made. Anyone deciding to use the focus group discussion method in their research should consult authoritative texts such as Krueger (1994), Krueger and King (1998), Morgan (1997, 1998) and Morgan and Krueger (1997/8), or undertake specialist training.

Diaries

Asking respondents to keep a daily account of their lives for a period of time might be seen as a more qualitative version of self-completion questionnaires. Here, instead of check boxes, selected people are asked to keep a record in their own words. In this method, although detailed instructions are given, there is no interviewer present to prompt or probe for further information or clarification, and you cannot be sure that others have not been consulted. Further, diaries usually require a considerable amount of extra work from respondents. Because of this you are likely to get either a high non-completion rate or only scant accounts from all but the very committed.

Although undertaken over forty years ago, Townsend's study of the lives of older people remains one of the best examples of the use of diaries in a mixed-method approach. Twenty of his 203 respondents were asked to keep diaries of their daily lives for a week. Of these, eight refused because they either could not write or just did not want to do it. The following excerpt illustrates the diary method.

Wednesday
   7.45 a.m.   We were up as I had to go to Doctor's with Dad. We just had a cup of tea and off we went at 9. Then we came home to Quaker Oats and bread and butter – that was 10 o'clock. I lit my fire, then cleared my kitchen up.
   11 a.m.   I went to the chemist first, then got my potatoes and a little piece of meat. I made a lot of it. I put it through the mincer with other little things and made a nice pie.
   1.0 p.m.   We had dinner and cup of tea and my daughter stayed with baby Carol. Nobody came after 6 o'clock, except my son John came with his wife to say good night before they went home from work.
   9.0 p.m.   We went to bed: I didn't feel so well with my back. (Townsend, 1963: 298)

Although this account appears very ordinary and unexceptional (and many accounts are), it is possible to identify information relating to various themes: diet; shopping trips; daily activities; responsibilities of carers; family visits. The analysis and interpretation of this kind of data are discussed in more detail in Chapter 10.

Special cases in interviewing

A potentially serious issue involved in collecting information by interviewing respondents is the power imbalance in the respondent/researcher relationship. This imbalance is rarely discussed in standard 'methods' texts, and is often only obliquely referred to in research reports. These power imbalances result from actual or perceived differences in social/professional status, culture, gender and age. It is important not only to be aware of these differences, but to attempt to minimize the possible sensitivities arising by using a suitable research design. In health needs assessments, you are most likely to face this power imbalance when studying an ethnically mixed community or when interviewing the medical profession.

If your study is of an ethnically mixed community, it is important that you include representatives from all of the ethnic groups in your community in the planning and design of the research. Each representative could then be responsible for their version of the questionnaire: its construction, piloting, data collection and processing. This approach has been adopted by Calderdale and Kirklees Health Authority in their health care planning consultations. Here members of minority ethnic groups have been trained to undertake their own projects with their own ethnic communities (Steering Group . . ., 1994, 1995). A further example of this approach is found in a study of the health needs of women from black and ethnic minority groups in Glasgow, undertaken by the Community Support Unit of the Glasgow Healthy City Project (Avan, 1995). In this project *informal group discussions* were held with eleven groups representing the range of 'class, religion, culture, age, etc.' found amongst the minority ethnic communities of Glasgow. In addition, one-to-one interviews were conducted with those who worked with these communities (for example, community workers, race relations officers and medical practitioners).

Interviews with medical practitioners should preferably be undertaken by a highly skilled interviewer or a fairly senior member of the research team. Thus, Neve, herself a GP, conducted the interviews with GPs in her community assessment (Neve, 1996). In contrast, the Bowling study of City and Hackney used a postal questionnaire to survey medical practitioners (Bowling, 1993).

Chapter summary

Asking questions of people is the most common method of getting information in social research. Unlike everyday 'asking', we use formal and *systematic techniques* to ask questions and record the answers that are given. These include constructing *topic lists*, *questionnaires* and *interview schedules* in such a way that we cover everything we need to know, in a manner appropriate to our research objectives.

In this chapter we saw how we can use *structured questionnaires* and *interview schedules* to obtain comparable answers in *social surveys*. Here the main goal is to obtain mainly standardized and limited information from a fairly large number of people. The resulting information is analysed using statistical techniques.

In contrast, when we want to explore people's experiences, feelings, meanings or understandings, we use less structured methods – *depth interviewing* or *diaries*. In these procedures the respondents talk or write about the research topics in their own way. Because the aim is depth rather than spread, research using these techniques involves only a small number of respondents. The resulting 'texts' or 'narratives' are analysed using qualitative methods.

Group discussions are used to find out about how opinions and attitudes are formed through social interaction. *Focus groups* are a special type of group discussion with highly formalized procedures. They have become very popular in many policy areas including consultative health projects and community profiling. However, focus groups should be used appropriately – to discover underlying issues and opinions, and the process of attitude formation – rather than as a cheaper substitute for a survey.

Exercise

The following questions were taken from actual self-completion questionnaires.

1 What is wrong with them?
2 Draft possible alternatives.

Question 1
Do you believe that increased violence and drug abuse is related to the higher level of unemployment?   ☐ Yes   ☐ No

Question 2
The loss of hedgerows in Britain is at an all time high with some 500,000 miles of hedgerow disappearing since 1947. Hedgerows are the habitat of shrubs and wildlife and their destruction, by intensive farming, is a direct attack on our environment. What do you think?

Question 3
How many journeys have you made in the last three months (not including this one) between the places named in Questions 5 and 6 by each of the following means of transport? PLEASE COUNT RETURN JOURNEYS AS **TWO** JOURNEYS

	1. 1st class daytime train	1	☐
	2. 1st class sleeper train	2	☐
	3. 1st class other overnight train	3	☐
PLEASE WRITE NUMBER OF	4. 2nd class daytime train	4	☐
JOURNEYS IN BOXES	5. 2nd class sleeper train	5	☐
PROVIDED IN RIGHT	6. 2nd class other overnight train	6	☐
HAND COLUMN	7. Bus/Coach	7	☐
	8. Car	8	☐
	9. Air	9	☐
	0. Other (please specify)	0	☐

CHAPTER 7

OBSERVATIONAL TECHNIQUES

To those new to social research, observation might appear to be the obvious method to use in a community study, since it is seen as closest to the methods we all use in our everyday lives when making sense of our social world. This is taken to imply that observation does not require learning new skills. Furthermore, because it is assumed that observation is a qualitative method, it is thought not to involve mastering any complicated statistics. However, this is not the case. Unlike our everyday observations, observation as a research tool is best seen as *systematic looking* and *listening*. Although it is used to obtain additional information in the face-to-face interviews discussed in Chapter 6, when used as the main or only data collection method it is extremely time consuming and requires considerable knowledge and skills. In addition, observation is not necessarily a qualitative technique since it can involve complex sampling, counting and coding procedures. Further, it is not the best technique to use if you want to discover people's opinions and attitudes, or to examine past and future events.

On the other hand, a large amount of information can be obtained about a community by undertaking observational studies. This is particularly so when they are used with other techniques as part of a mixed-method approach. In this chapter, we will examine the various types of observation, the methods of recording observational data, and the advantages, limitations and dangers of the method.

Sampling and gaining entry

It is impossible to observe the whole social life of a community, however small it is. Even in a small interest-based group such as a women's group that comes together in a single location, time constraints and multiple interactions limit what can be simultaneously observed and recorded: you cannot see everything that is going on at once. In larger communities these constraints are compounded by both population size and multiple locations. Thus, decisions have to be made about who, where, what and when to observe – you have to sample.

Your selection will, of course, be determined by the nature of your study: your definition of health, whose health etc. Random sampling (discussed in Chapter 5) could be used to select, for example, which clubs and groups to study or at what times to observe. Alternatively, and more usually, purposive sampling is used. Here, researchers select what they think are the most appropriate settings and groups. Because of the bias this introduces, purposive sampling is often combined with what is termed *theoretical sampling*.

In theoretical sampling, findings from previous observations are tested out on other groups in order to investigate how generalizable they are. This process is continued until all relevant categories have been studied and *theoretical saturation* is reached. For example, you may find that large trucks were causing severe problems for people crossing a particular road. You would then test this by observing at different time periods and/or in different roads. You might also investigate whether different types of people were equally affected, or whether other types of vehicles caused similar problems, and so on.

Observations in public places are fairly unproblematic in terms of access, although it is advisable to inform the police. In closed settings such as clubs and meeting places, GPs' waiting rooms and other institutional locations, it is necessary to obtain permission to carry out the research. In medical settings you will need to approach the local *medical ethics committee*, in addition to the research vetting procedures of your own organization. You will also need to gain the permission and support of those in charge of the particular setting. These *gatekeepers* are likely to have an important impact on – and thus bias – your research in several ways. First, by restricting access they can control who, what, when and where you are able to carry out your observations. Second, their interpretation of what you are studying will influence what they think you should see. Third, if they introduce you to the group, their interpretation of your research is likely to influence how the group behaves in your presence. Finally, as your sponsor, their position in relation to the group will affect how members of the group perceive your position and their relationship with you.

The structure of observation

Observation as a technique of social research differs from the naturalistic *looking* and *listening* that we use in our ordinary lives, where the processes of seeing and hearing are passive. Here, unless we are especially looking for something or someone, the visual images and sounds that we acquire are taken for granted, and we only actively notice the unusual. This does not mean that we go around bumping into people or objects, rather we respond (by avoiding, for example) without consciously seeing. For instance, can you remember how many people you *saw* when you last walked down a busy street? More importantly, can you describe them, who they were with, what they were doing, and what were they saying? In contrast, observation as a research tool is *active* looking and listening: seeing, noticing, hearing and *recording*. In this respect, it is similar to the process that visual artists use to see and record the forms of the subjects of their art works. This process is *structured* and *systematic*.

The degree of structure is determined by the nature of your research. First, you will need to prepare a topic list based on your knowledge of the aspects that you are interested in. This might be fairly specific, like those drawn up before designing a questionnaire. For example, you might be interested in examining environmental pollution in a particular area. Here, you would first define what you meant by environmental pollution and draw up a list of topics based upon this (noxious gases; rubbish; dog fouling; unsightly buildings; traffic noise; and so on). This list might be further refined by reference to particular days and times of day, specific sites within the area, individuals and groups responsible etc. You would then devise a method for measuring and recording these by observation rather than by questioning.

Alternatively, you might be interested in a topic on which there is little previous information or in a more general study of a particular community. Here, your research would be more exploratory in nature and your topic list less detailed – like in semi-/un-structured interviewing discussed in Chapter 6. In this case, the initial observations would be used to guide subsequent ones and theoretical sampling is likely to be used. Clearly, this type of observation requires the observer to be far more knowledgeable about the topic and more highly skilled and experienced in the techniques of observation than is necessary in a structured study.

Although many research methods textbooks classify observation as a qualitative method, it is not necessarily so. As in laboratory experiments, social activities can be measured or, at least, counted using observational methods. The structured example given above would be likely to include a considerable amount of quantitative data about the number of vehicles, illegal dumps, dog droppings, litter bins, and decibel readings, for instance. Other, more sophisticated, measurements have been used for many years to study small group interactions based on techniques developed in the late 1940s (Bales, 1950).

Non-participant observation

Observational studies in which the researcher's role is to record what is seen and heard without otherwise taking part in any activities is termed *non-participant observation*. This type of observation includes both observations of small group activities and what is often called 'the community walk' or 'casing the joint'. Here, those being studied may have previously been informed about the research – the observation is *overt* – or they may not (*covert* observation). Both types have important consequences for the research.

In overt observation, there is the risk of error and bias being introduced by the *research effect*. Here there is a high probability that those who are observed will behave differently because they know that they are being observed. Covert observation, on the other hand, is regarded by many researchers as unethical because it does not comply with the principle of informed consent (see Chapter 1). Others would argue that research is ethical so long as it does not harm anyone and that no one is identifiable in any reports arising from the research. Here, there is a tendency to use the term *unobtrusive* rather than covert – probably because it sounds less like snooping!

Perhaps the most familiar example of non-participant observation that you will encounter in community needs assessments is the community walk. There are few explicit descriptions of this in health literature but it underlies much of the more recent community-oriented fieldwork (see, for example, Murray and Graham, 1995; Lapthorne, 1996). This form of observation is usually undertaken early in a study, as a preliminary or exploratory stage. Here, the researchers 'case the joint' to get a feel of the physical surroundings and how they impact on the social life of the community. It can also be used as part of a mixed-method approach – to add more depth to a survey, for example. Before undertaking this type of study you would, of course, need to draw up a topic list and decide how to record your observations. This list might include a count of the number and range of shops and who uses them; study traffic flows and identify dangerous crossing points or high levels of exhaust emission; and inspect play areas and parks for evidence of litter, broken glass and dog droppings. In the work place, there may be dangerous machinery, steps, and so on that could be recorded or you might observe what people eat at meal breaks. In addition, you might watch and listen to what people say in informal meetings, in local shops, pubs, at vending machines, and at local clinics or committee meetings.

In health needs assessments of communities you will encounter studies that use non-participatory observations of small groups less often, since you are most likely to be participating in them in some way: as a member, or having a professional involvement. In the medical setting this type of research is often undertaken as a preliminary and is rarely reported. For example, in their study of hospital visiting, Abbott and Payne used researchers to stand outside of the wards at various times in order to observe visitors' activities before the interviewing stage of the research (Abbott and Payne, 1992; Payne, 1998). Another example of this method from the wider 'health' field is Warren's study of home helps in Salford. Here, the method was combined with group discussions (Warren, 1990).

Participant observation

When researchers undertake participant observation they attempt to study a community or group from the inside by *participating* in its social life. Here, they would adopt a role within the group: as a new resident, patient, colleague or member. Clearly, the role would need to be appropriate. For example, researchers in their twenties would not join an Over-Sixties club as members, although they might become helpers. Participant observation is usually covert. This approach avoids the problems of researcher bias associated with overt observation, since members of the group do not know that they are being studied.

However, in participant observation a researcher not only has to face the ethical problem of breaching the principle of informed consent, but also other sources of bias are introduced. First, the role adopted by the researcher will influence what can be observed. Unlike the overt researcher, a participant observer cannot be a 'researcher' who is able to move around various different groups to get an overall picture. Thus, once you join a group as a patient, say, you cannot become a staff member or vice versa. Second, by being a participant you will be expected to be *actively* involved in the life of the group and, however much you attempt to behave neutrally, your actions and opinions are likely to influence the group. Third, not only should your observations be unobtrusive but the recording of them should be done surreptitiously. This often necessitates making notes after the event when memory error is likely to be a significant biasing factor. Finally, all participant observers face the problem of *going native*. 'Going native' is the term used to describe situations in which researchers become so immersed in the adopted role that they actually become part of the group and cease to be researchers.

Participant observation has been most successfully used in the many community studies undertaken, particularly in the 1950s, 1960s and 1970s, by anthropologists and sociologists who usually lived in the community that they were studying (see, for instance, Bell and Newby, 1971; Cohen, 1982; Payne, 1996). Although often used covertly, this method was frequently combined with depth interviewing and surveys as part of a mixed-method approach to the study of various aspects of community life. Here, the work of the Institute of Community Studies which was based in the East End of London during the 1950s, is a prime example (Townsend, 1963; Young and Willmott, 1957).

Within the health field, research using participant observation has been concentrated principally in institutional settings and on professional training or work. Lately, it has also been employed as part of the mixed-method Rapid Appraisal approach, discussed in Chapter 8. Among recent reports, Kirkham's description of her overt study of staff/patient communication on a labour ward is, perhaps, one of the most clear accounts of the method (Kirkham, 1992). Here, not only does she discuss the theoretical and methodological justification of her approach, but also some of the practical and ethical problems that she faced while undertaking the study.

Methods of recording observational data

The methods used to record observational data are very much determined by the degree of structure, the obtrusiveness of the design and the ingenuity of the researcher. However, whatever type of observational method is used, it is important to decide at the planning stage of the project what data to record and how to record them. These methods can then be tested by piloting. The usual recording techniques are the pro-forma, the notebook and/or dictaphone, the audio recorder, the still camera and the video recorder.

A highly structured observational study might use a pro-forma, similar to a pre-coded questionnaire. In such cases, the pre-coding may allow for ticks and other symbols in addition to the usual alphanumeric codes (see, for instance, Bales, 1950; Bell, 1987). Usually, however, you are more likely to record your observations verbatim or by personal notations, setting down whatever happens in a given situation, including your own feelings and interpretations. This might be impossible in covert observation. Here, you might be able to make some brief notes that would be expanded and written up or dictated later. If you are planning to write up your observations after they have been made, you should restrict the length of each observational event to a time period that allows for your total recall of events. Further, it is important to avoid speaking to anyone about the observations until you have recorded them, because your account of the observations is likely to be affected by this encounter.

As well as recording your observations, you should keep a *research diary* or *journal*. Here, all your thoughts, experiences and any ideas about the research are recorded for later scrutiny and analysis. Through this process of *reflexive subjectivity*, you can become aware of how your own biases, perspectives and actions may influence the research. The following extract from a research journal illustrates how reflexivity is recorded.

> I think my enthusiasm for the problems of integration (i.e. my desire for it to work) is blinding me to the real problems of the teachers who are stymied by overwork and administrative responsibilities and can no longer see how it can work. I feel frustrated with their depressed attitudes – suspect most regard people with disabilities as a waste of time and effort in this economic climate. I think I'll pull out of schools for a bit and go back to interviewing parents and observing and interviewing in institutions. (Grbich, 1999: 90)

Visual recordings

The recording of overt observations can include videos and photography to supplement your note-taking or as data in their own right. Both these methods can provide very rich data and are particularly useful when you are presenting your results. Before using a still camera or camcorder you must, of course, ensure that everyone is agreeable. Complete informed consent is, however, virtually impossible in a busy street or other public place. Here, common sense and sensitivity are important, especially with regard to the subsequent use of the images in any presentation.

In addition to ethical considerations, it is important to be aware that visual images are no more objective than more traditional observations. Visual images are the result of the subjective selectivity of the person recording them, and your reasons for selecting to record events should be noted in your research diary. Further, people often behave differently when they know that they are being filmed. However, if filming can be done unobtrusively – but with consent – people do get used to it: for instance, we tend to take for granted the CCTV cameras in shops and town centres. Examples of using video cameras in health research include studies of hospital interactions undertaken by Bottoroff (1994) and Brooker (1993). In the Bottoroff study of nurse–patient interactions, cameras were installed a month before the start of data collection so that participants could get used to them being there. The cameras were then monitored from a separate office and observations made from them at the time. These observations were complemented by interviews (Grbich, 1999). In contrast, Brooker's study of nurse–visitor interaction and the negotiation of space used a video camera in a hospital ward as the primary method of data collection. Here, observations were made from the recorded video tape afterwards (Harrison, 1996).

Before using either still or videos cameras, you should make sure that you are technically competent in their use. This is particularly so when using a video camera. Here, you need to have some knowledge of the general principles of filming, in addition to knowing how to operate it. First, you should ensure that you get the correct light balance. Artificial lighting is different from outdoor natural lighting, and very strange results can be achieved if the wrong setting is selected. Second, you should make sure that you can hold the camera steady, especially when zooming or panning. Here, a tripod, although expensive, is valuable. Third, do not move the camera or your position too often – let what you are filming move, not you. You should also take longer lengths of an event or object than you think you will need, particularly if you are going to edit the tape. Finally, you should make a story board either before you record or before you edit. Editing, itself, can take a considerable time, and you should allow for this in your research plan.

When using a video, and in any subsequent editing, you should be aware that you are *selecting* events and cases and *constructing* a story. In doing this, it is important to determine whether you are choosing 'good' or 'typical' shots. Further, you will need to decide whether you will sequence the 'story' in the order in which it occurred naturally (including the mundane bits!) or re-order it and select the more 'dramatic' events. These decisions should all be recorded in your diary.

Photographs are far easier and cheaper to take and use than video. In addition to taking photographs yourself, you might consider asking different groups or individuals to make their own photographic record. These visual accounts can provide very rich data on personal visions that cannot be collected by any other method. Also, they could be exhibited as both a visual history of the area or group and as a focus and 'memory jogger' for oral accounts of community life. Thus, images can be both used as a method of *recording* events and people and as an aid to *data collection and interpretation*. Again, as with video recordings, you should be aware of the processes of selection and construction of events.

These visual methods are particularly appropriate for involving children and teenagers in your study. This approach was adopted by Schratz and Steiner-Löffler (1998) in a primary school evaluation project in Austria. Pupils were divided into groups of four or five and asked to make a visual record of those places in the school that they felt good about and those that they thought were bad. After discussion, the groups took photographs of their selected spaces. Each group then made a series of collages (images made from combining fragments of other images) of their work with explanations of their feelings. This approach could easily be adapted to discover what children think is good or bad about their community for instance.

This method might also include drawings and paintings. The World Health Organization's *Healthy Cities Project Report* (Tsouros, 1990) includes reproductions from a drawing and painting competition for children in Pécs, Hungary on the theme of 'health and my city'. The illustrations include ideas about the environment, sport and leisure, housing and community activities. Interestingly, none of the art works included depict any images of death or disease. Other non-health related examples include exhibitions of children's art from Northern Ireland and Bosnia.

The *Draw and Write* technique used by the Health Education Authority (HEA) for school health education programmes was developed from research on language development (Wetton and McWhirter, 1998). In the ensuing work commissioned by the HEA, children were asked to make annotated drawings of what they did to make and keep themselves healthy. Although the analysis was mainly of the written accounts, later analysis of the drawings showed children to have a broad definition of health. Here

> health is not limited to physical aspects but includes mental and emotional health . . . Those images where people were not smiling carried written health warnings such as don't smoke, don't take drugs or beware of out of date food . . . Although food and exercise were the largest categories of response, children stressed the social aspects of being healthy – having a home, a family and friends, playing and working hard, as well as environmental health. (Wetton and McWhirter, 1998: 274)

Again, as with the Austrian example discussed above, this approach could be adapted for a study of community health needs.

Observational skills

The particular features of observation require that the researcher has a wider range of skills than those needed for asking questions. This is especially so for semi- or unstructured participant observation. Here, the researcher normally works alone and, thus, has sole responsibility for data collection. This requires the same unbiased or reflexive approach, adaptability, flexibility, recording accuracy and ability to 'get on with others' as the interviewer role. In addition, however, a more thorough knowledge of the topic and an ability to observe and record multiple activities is needed.

Adaptability and flexibility are required when one is faced with any unforeseen problems that arise, both technical and topic related. The researcher must attempt to deal with such events in a way that does not prejudice the research or bias the findings. For example, by taking sides in a dispute or expressing a particular opinion when asked, a researcher is likely to be seen as being associated with one specific group rather than another and, thus, close off future research possibilities. However,

to be seen *not* to be taking any action can also work against you. Further, if things do not happen as the preliminary investigations have suggested, the research should be adapted to allow for this.

It is highly likely that a researcher may have to record simultaneous events during fieldwork. People cannot be asked to repeat actions because they were missed. This requires being able to be creative in the use of shorthand-like symbols and, inevitably, being selective. In making choices about what to record, a researcher must make decisions about the relevance of events to the central research topic. Thus, one researcher records in her notes:

> One of the problems all during today has been the vast input of possible information, and not knowing how to select it. I'd already decided that for the first couple of days I'd concentrate on my own socialization, the acquiring of the routine, learning about the ward and so on to be able to write down the timetable of the nursing day, but even so. (James, 1992: 14)

This type of research not only requires the researcher to record what is seen and heard but, through theoretical sampling and self-questioning, to develop, test and refine ideas that arise from the observations themselves. This process should also be recorded so that as full a processual account as possible is achieved. These accounts can then be scrutinized during post-fieldwork analysis for possible sources of bias etc.

Clearly these abilities and attributes are only acquired through practice and experience. No one new to research should, or would be expected to, undertake a major participant observation study without guidance and training from an experienced practitioner. However, it would be possible for them to undertake the more structured forms of observation that are used in 'the community walk', for example, where they are accompanied by more experienced researchers.

Chapter summary

Observational studies can provide extremely rich data that are impossible to collect using any other technique. However, they should not be used indiscriminately since there are certain types of information that cannot be obtained using observation alone: past and future events, feelings, opinions and attitudes, and private domestic behaviour. Further, the many potential sources of bias, particularly when *participant* observations are undertaken by only one researcher, create problems relating to the reliability of the findings: if repeated by someone else, would the findings be similar? Finally, *covert* observation raises serious *ethical issues* concerning the principle of *informed consent*. For this reason, many researchers will undertake observational studies only if those to be observed are aware of the study and have given their consent.

Exercise

For this exercise, you should choose a partner and inform the police about your study.

1   Each select a small area comprising a few streets.
2   Draw up a list of topics relating to environmental factors that affect people's health.
3   Decide how these can be measured using observational techniques.
4   Undertake observations in your selected area using the resulting list, but do not discuss them until they are recorded.
5   Compare your findings.

CHAPTER 8

EXISTING PROCEDURES AND EVALUATIONS

The previous three chapters have discussed the main techniques that researchers use to collect new information about various aspects of social life. These methods, particularly the more quantitative ones, have been used in the health field for many years. More recently, changes within the NHS itself, the need to listen to 'local voices', for example, and a growing concern with the wider socio-economic aspects of health, have led to a proliferation of new approaches, tools and packages that offer competing methods of assessing health and health status. Thus, rather than devise your research project from scratch, it would appear sensible where possible to use one or more of these existing procedures. This chapter will begin by an examination of these.

These procedures can be broadly divided into the highly structured *health status profiles* and *indices*, and the more diverse *community profiling* methods. Although the first group are not appropriate to use as the *only* method of assessing community health needs, they could be combined with other techniques in a mixed-method approach. In contrast, some of the community profiling procedures have been used as a main method in health assessments. Before using these techniques, however, it is important to decide on their *applicability* to your study and to assess their *validity* and *reliability*.

The chapter then looks at investigations over time. In assessing health needs we not only need appropriate, valid and reliable methods but we also have to decide on a time framework for the assessment: should it be a one-off time-specific study or should the community or group be studied over a longer period? *Longitudinal* or *panel* studies have been used successfully for many years to investigate different aspects of health but, because of financial constraints, have only very recently been used in community profiling. The advantages and limitations of this method will be discussed with reference to both national and local examples. Finally, we will examine the different approaches to, and types of, *evaluation*. These include both parallel and post-hoc evaluative research.

Reviewing existing procedures

Using an existing procedure in your project rather than developing your own research design can save a considerable amount of time and effort. However, it is important that such procedures are *appropriate* or *applicable* to your particular study. In assessing their suitability you should discover whether these procedures answer your research questions: what definition of health is implied; what type of population do they cover; what range of topics are included, and in what detail? You should also find out what methods of data collection and analysis are needed since these might be beyond your capabilities in terms of personnel, skills and other resources. In addition to the applicability of a procedure you will also need to investigate its *validity* and *reliability*. These are discussed in Chapter 3.

Health status profiles and indices

Health status profiles and indices include questionnaires and scaling methods designed to measure general levels of health, outcome measures of specific diseases and treatments, and those that aim to assess health related quality of life (HRQL). Detailed descriptions of these (including the three we shall look at as most relevant to health needs assessments) are given in Bowling (1997), which is the best current text on this topic. Here, she classifies them into five broad categories: the measurement of function ability; broader measures of health status; measures of psychological well being; measurements of social networks and social support; and measures of life satisfaction and morale. A full discussion of these devices is beyond the scope of this book since they are, in the main, measures of individual health status for use in clinical assessments. However, three techniques that have been used in community-based research are *Townsend's Disability Scale*, the *Nottingham Health Profile* and the *Short Form-36* (and 12).

Townsend's Disability Scale

This disability scale has been used in various different forms for many studies of elderly people in the UK (for instance, Bond and Carstairs, 1982; Bowling et al., 1988; Sainsbury, 1973; Townsend, 1962, 1979). Although primarily used to study disability in older people, it does have more general application and can be used in self-completion and interview surveys. Its main advantage is that it is relatively short and easy to complete.

The questionnaire consists of a list of everyday tasks (for example, washing, dressing, preparing a meal, climbing stairs, shopping, housework) that respondents are asked to rate according to the level of difficulty they have in undertaking them. These ratings were originally scored on a scale of 0–3, but the range was increased to 0–5 in some modified versions. The zero means 'no difficulty' in all versions, and the higher values are equated with increasing difficulty. The individual scores are then added together to give an overall disability measure.

In her evaluation, Bowling found that the original index had been subject to only minimal testing. Further, citing Sainsbury (1973), she found that the tasks had been selected subjectively. Validity and reliability testing undertaken on later modifications of the scale show fairly good correlations with the Nottingham Health Profile (see below) and physical health problems (Bowling, 1997: 28–9).

The Nottingham Health Profile (NHP)

This questionnaire was designed in the early 1980s by Hunt and her colleagues in Nottingham (Hunt et al., 1986) to reflect wider definitions of health than those based on a medical/disease model. The final questions were derived from the results of a large survey of the general public about the ways in which illness affects behaviour. The first section of the questionnaire consists of 38 questions requiring simple Yes/No answers. These questions cover six broad dimensions of health: mobility, pain, energy, sleep, emotions, and social isolation. The second part goes on to ask about the effects of a person's health on seven areas of life: work, housework, social, family, sex, interests/hobbies, and holidays. Again the questions only require simple Yes/No answers. Table 8.1 gives examples of the types of statements included.

A scoring system has been devised for Part 1 so that each of the six dimension can range from 0 ('no' to all) to 100 ('yes' to all). Average scores for general and specific population groups are available for comparison. Full details of the questionnaire and the scoring system are given in Hunt et al. (1986). Permission to use the form has to be obtained from the authors although no charge is made. The NHP is a very easy, quick and cheap method to use, but it has been found to be poor at identifying mild illness and is a measure of disease and impairment rather than health.

The NHP was included as part of a larger questionnaire used by Murray and Graham (1995) in their study of the Dumbiedykes estate in Edinburgh. This study used a range of methods and aimed not only to

Table 8.1 *Sample statements from the Nottingham Health Profile*

I can only walk about indoors
I find it hard to bend
Everything is an effort
Worry is keeping me awake at night
I feel there is nobody I am close to

---

identify the health needs of the residents but also to compare the results obtained from the different methods. They found that the NHP identified higher rates of chronic illness than GP records, and residents scored far worse than expected on each sub-scale. Generally the researchers found that the NHP provided useful information as part of a mixed-method approach.

In discussing the validity and reliability of this questionnaire, Bowling found that the Nottingham Health Profile had a 'fairly high level of reliability', was a good discriminator between different health states, and was sensitive to health changes over time. However, it is 'a negative measure of health' and, as such, it does not test for all disabilities and disorders: sight and anorexia, for example. Because of these limitations, the Nottingham Health Profile would be of limited value in a community health needs assessment.

Short Form-36/12 (SF-36; SF-12)

In contrast to NHP, Short Form-36 was originally developed in America for use by health insurance companies and has been adapted for British use: for example, 'full of pep' becomes 'full of life' (Brazier et al., 1992). SF-36 consists of 35 questions that measure three broad aspects of health: function, well being, and overall health. A further question asks about current health compared with a year ago. A shortened version (Short Form-12) has recently been developed in Boston. Both have been found to be fairly good methods of assessing the results of treatments and as measures of general health status. Examples of the questions are given in Table 8.2. The questionnaires are still being evaluated for use in the UK and have been the subject of lengthy correspondence in the *British Medical Journal* (see, especially, issues for 1993 and 1994). For full details of the validity and reliability tests see Bowling (1997: 59–60).

One such evaluation was carried out by a team from Aberdeen University. Their investigation involved the administration of the questionnaire to a sample of GP patients in the Grampian Region. The responses of those who were identified as suffering from four common

Table 8.2. *Examples of questions from Short Form-36*

Compared to **one year ago**, how would you rate your health in general **now?**
  Much better than one year ago
  Somewhat better than one year ago
  About the same
  Somewhat worse than one year ago
  Much worse than one year ago

During the **past 4 weeks**, how much did **pain** interfere with your normal work (including work both outside the home and housework)?
  Not at all
  A little bit
  Moderately
  Quite a bit
  Extremely

complaints were compared with a general sample from the population of the Region. They found that the SF-36 was a consistent and valid measure of health status and was easily completed by respondents (Garrett et al., 1993).

However, it is based on the narrow disease model of health rather than the wider 'new public health' definition and is therefore of limited use for a community-based approach. Like the NHP, it is probably best used as part of a mixed-method approach. Again, as with the NHP, SF-36 and SF-12 are free but permission must be obtained from: Dr John E. Ware, Jr, The Health Institute, New England Medical Center Hospital, NEMCH Box 345, 750 Washington Street, Boston, Ma 02111, USA.

Community profiling procedures

The term 'community profile' covers a wide range of research procedures that have been used to obtain mainly quantitative information to inform public policy or to evaluate policy initiatives. In these studies 'a community' usually means a small locality-based group. There are many examples of these profiles variously undertaken by statutory bodies, pressure groups and communities themselves. However, many of them remain unpublished, although subsequent reports can be obtained from some of the more recent studies. Details are given in Hawtin et al. (1994) and Laughlin and Black (1995).

Three of the most widely known or used procedures are discussed in this section. These are *Rapid Appraisal*, an increasingly popular approach in community health needs assessment, *Priority Search*, a package used by many Healthy City initiatives, and *Compass*, a more general community profiling software package developed from the rural profiling methods of *Village Appraisal*.

Rapid Appraisal (RA)

Rapid Appraisal uses a mixed-method approach adapted from community profiling techniques used in Third World countries. It uses three of the methods discussed in previous chapters to obtain an overall view of a (usually) locality-based community. These are:

- The construction of a profile from existing statistical and documentary sources.
- Direct observations in the community.
- Interviews and group discussions with 'key informants' (people who work in a professional capacity in the community, community representatives and other prominent locals: for example, shopkeepers).

The information collected is categorized as an 'information pyramid' consisting of four layers, further divided into nine broad areas. These are shown in Figure 8.1.

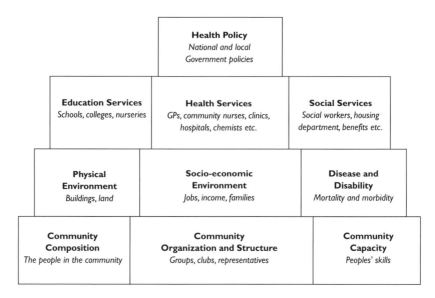

Figure 8.1 *Example of a Rapid Appraisal information pyramid*

This method is increasing in popularity. Examples of its use can be found in studies of Dumbiedykes (Murray and Graham, 1995), Merseyside, Northern Ireland, Stoke and London (Ong and Humphris, 1994). It was also used in the Devonport Initiative in Plymouth (Lapthorne, 1996). As its name suggests, it is a fairly fast method of obtaining information – the Dumbiedykes study took five community professionals, working four hours a day on average, three months to collect – and provides a broad range of information about the community.

Its main weakness is its reliance on key informants providing the detailed qualitative information. This is highlighted as a weakness in *Local Voices* (NHS Management Executive, 1992). As discussed in Chapter 6, key informants do not necessarily represent the whole range of attitudes and opinions in the community. If used with a wider survey, *Rapid Appraisal* could form the basis for a thorough assessment of a locality-based community. Further, the nine broad categories of information provide a sound framework for establishing a project and might be used as a basis for other methods.

Priority Search

This is more clearly a 'package' than the methods previously discussed in this chapter. *Priority Search* is a computerized questionnaire method developed in the late 1980s by a group working within Sheffield City Council. It is based on the theory that there are 'underlying consistencies in the way we see, or construct, the world' (Priority Search, 1994: Appendix (v)). The *Priority Search* method attempts to uncover these.

The first stage is to identify a general question that can be used as the basis for one or more focus groups. Examples of this include 'What would improve your health, happiness and well being?' and 'What would make Bootle a better place to live in?' (Priority Search, 1992, 1994). Focus groups are then held with people drawn from a sample of the population to be surveyed. The statements made in the focus groups in answer to the general question are then used to form the basis of a questionnaire. This questionnaire repeats the general question but then provides a list of alternative statements. Respondents are asked to compare each statement with another one using a sliding scale of fifty circles (see Figure 8.2). Individual statements are included three times, each time being compared with a different statement. This provides for a full range of alternatives to be made.

The questionnaires are then processed and analysed using a technique called *Principal Component Analysis*. This is a statistical method that groups all of the answers and preferences into a smaller number of underlying attitudes: for example, bullying and racism, safer streets

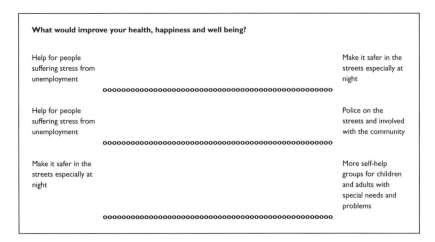

Figure 8.2 *Example of a Priority Search comparison scale* (from the Thamesdown survey, Priority Search, 1994)

and policing are all statements about security; more nurseries, play areas and teenage venues are all about child care.

Although the commissioning researchers would decide on the general question and local people might be involved in interviewing, the *Priority Search* team would have to be employed to undertake the focus groups, design and analyse the questionnaire and prepare the final report. They stress that their charges are flexible and can be open to negotiation. Local 'experts' could also be used for some of the stages. Their address is: Priority Focus, Room G9, Old Town Hall, Surrey Street, Sheffield, S1 2HH. Alternatively, an approximation of this method could possibly be carried out locally at a lower cost.

Compass community profiling software

Compass is a computer package that can be used to manage your project, questionnaire design, data processing and analysis. The package was developed jointly by the Countryside Community Research Unit, Cheltenham and the Policy Research Institute, Leeds. It is based on the *Village Appraisal* package developed by the Cheltenham group to assist in rural community studies. These packages are protected by copyright. Local experts could help you use them, but the software has to be obtained from the authors: Compass Sales, Policy Research Institute, 16 Queen Square, Leeds, LS2 8AJ.

The package is a general community profiling tool consisting of over 400 pre-written questions. These cover a range of topics including housing, health, employment, income, education, training, and environment. Users can select from this list and/or add their own questions. The questions selected are then used to produce a standard form for a self-completion or interview survey. The package will also generate a data entry form that can be used to input responses, and a statistical analysis component to provide tables, charts and graphs. The package is very reasonably priced (determined by the type of organization) and comes with full documentation. In addition, the group will arrange a half-day, on-site introductory course.

Because of the flexibility of the questionnaire, the range of components and the costs, this package would appear to be a good solution for researchers who either do not have the time or necessary skills to produce their own questionnaire. Like the other methods discussed, however, unless you 'contract out' your project, you will still need to carry out preliminary research, sampling, print questionnaires, interviewing, data input and report writing. The author was only able to discover one community health project that had used the software – in Barne Barton, Plymouth (Maconachie, 1997). Thus, the package has not been used sufficiently for any meaningful evaluation of its validity or reliability to be made.

Longitudinal studies

The examples we have discussed so far have been one-off studies that have investigated various aspects of health at a particular point in time. These study designs are more than adequate for meeting the aims of most of the projects that you might undertake in health needs assessment research. However, because they are 'snapshots' (taken at *one point in time*), they do not provide information about changes that occur *over time*. Even life history interviews are subject to memory error and falsifications that usually cannot be checked. Instead, the most appropriate method for studying temporal events is the *longitudinal* or *panel* study. This can be broadly defined as a study of the same sample of individuals on at least two occasions. Most examples, however, collect information more frequently than this, often over a period of many years.

In the medical setting you are most likely to come across this approach in controlled trials, child development studies or case records. Perhaps the most famous studies in the UK are the *Population Investigation Committee*, the *National Child Development Study* and the *British*

Cohort Study using 1946, 1958 and 1970 birth cohorts respectively. The data from these studies have provided important research findings in the fields of public health and education (Douglas, 1981). Another well-known example is the *Whitehall Study*. This study has traced the health of 17,000 male civil servants since 1967 (see, for instance, Marmot et al., 1984; Marmot and Theorell, 1988; Marmot et al., 1991). In addition to such large scale national studies, panels have been used to study people's opinions about aspects of health service provision (McHarg, 1996) and priorities in health (Richardson and Bowie, 1995). In the wider social and market research fields, longitudinal studies have been mainly confined to educational research, audience research and voting behaviour panels. Here, Wall and Williams's (1970) text remains one of the best accounts.

Since 1971, the Office of National Statistics (ONS) has linked vital registration records (births and deaths) to the Census records of one per cent of the population of England and Wales (Goldblatt, 1990; Harding, 1995). This project, known to most researchers as 'the LS' ('the Longitudinal Study'), is accessible through a central team now located at the London University Institute of Education (LS User Support Programme, Centre for Longitudinal Studies (CLS), Institute of Education (6th Floor), 20 Bedford Way, London WC1H 0AL). The LS provides a core data-set on which a variety of studies have been based. Its growing popularity comes from the fact that, within sensible constraints about anonymity and confidentiality, a cohort of people can be traced through the 1971, 1981, 1991 – and in due course 2001 – Censuses. When individuals drop out over time (a problem for all longitudinal analysis) there is a mechanism for replacing them. Socio-economic circumstances can be connected to medical records, and a number of special studies are also linked: for instance the Carstairs deprivation score (Carstairs and Morris, 1989), or older data on pollution, water quality and climate from the British Regional Heart Study (Pocock et al., 1980). This resource is being used to explore a variety of topics, including area deprivation and low birthweight, mortality and long-term illness rates, poverty and household composition, and teenage pregnancies (ONS/CLS, 1998).

Although the LS was not originally intended for very local studies, it may be possible to draw on it for this purpose. It has data on the areas in which its members live and have lived at the Census times, classified into types by local demography, housing conditions, household make-up, and employment circumstances. In most cases, it can produce data by Travel to Work Areas, local authority areas, wards and enumeration districts. It may thus be possible to use data already collected in the LS sample, either instead of new data collection, or to compare with your own findings.

Despite the advantages of providing change data, there are five main problems with undertaking new local longitudinal studies. Most obviously, the costs of the research are far higher than one-off studies. These costs include not only the direct costs of data collection and processing on more than one occasion, but also those involved with maintaining contact with respondents over a period of years, with continuity of staffing, and physical resources. And very few grant-giving bodies are likely to guarantee monies for more than five years.

Second, there are major problems involved with recruitment. Initially, researchers have to persuade prospective respondents – or their parents – that there is value (to them and/or society) in making a commitment to be studied over a period of years. Even when this is forthcoming, follow-up problems arise relating to maintaining contact, motivation and cooperation. Over time, migration, deaths, drop-outs and non-contacts increase non-response rates and, thus, reduce the representativeness of the sample.

A third problem relates to the issue of relevance. Data that were relevant to researchers at the start of a study may be obsolete years later, or currently important data may not have been collected. Hence, many longitudinal studies become costly 'white elephants', providing decreasing research benefits. Related to this is the problem of staff continuity. Although good documentation, briefing and training may reduce problems caused by staff turnover, research interests and popularity do change over time, with consequent effects on the study. Finally, longitudinal studies are faced with the problem of what is often called *'the Hawthorne effect'* in which respondents become conditioned to being studied and behave differently. Obviously this conditioning leads to the introduction of various sources of incalculable bias.

Despite these problems, it is possible to undertake small panel studies over a short time scale that provide useful data. For example, Calderdale and Kirklees Health Authority have used 'standing panels' drawn from both the general population and particular minority ethnic groups. These panels are sent self-completion questionnaires three times a year to obtain their opinions on health and local authority services. To maintain cooperation, group discussions are held and newsletters sent to provide feedback reports (McHarg, 1996).

A further example of the use of this approach in the health field is Gordon's study of depressed women. This study is a typical *controlled trial* in which women were allocated to one of two groups – experimental and control. Psychological tests to assess level of depression were carried out on both groups at the beginning and end of the trial period. Those in the experimental group undertook weekly group therapy discussion sessions over a period of 14 weeks. Those in the control group had no contact. Test results were compared to assess the effects of the group sessions (Gordon, 1992).

Evaluations

Evaluative research is undertaken to assess the *worth* of something. In the health field this 'something' could be a treatment, a programme, a policy or a project. Social evaluation is not a method or technique like the social survey or participant observation. It is a particular type of applied social research that might employ any or all of the research methods discussed in this book.

This kind of research focuses on measurements (numeric or descriptive) of *inputs*, *outputs* and *processes*: it studies *change*. At their most basic, evaluations replicate the classic scientific experimental method or 'OXO'. Here, units are observed ('O') before and after something ('X') is done to them, and the observed measures are compared and evaluated. It is fairly easy, in the laboratory setting, to make sure that factors other than 'X' are not introduced between the two observation points. However, when dealing with people and social activities we cannot control the variables in the same way and, therefore, different approaches are needed.

The familiar and well-documented clinical research method of *randomized controlled trials* was developed to minimize the influence of extraneous factors. This approach matches people on certain characteristics (age, gender, etc.) and randomly allocates the resulting *matched pairs* to one of two groups: the experimental and the control. Tests ('O') are then undertaken, treatment ('X') is given to the experimental group, and further tests ('O') are carried out. The results are then analysed and an evaluation of the treatment is made. Gordon's study of depressed women, discussed in the previous section, is one example of this method (Gordon, 1992). This approach, however, has limited application for studies of the health needs of communities, although it might be used for specific projects on diet, smoking or exercise, for example. Detailed descriptions of this method are given in most standard textbooks on medical research (see, for instance, Shepperd et al., 1997). The method is critically evaluated in Pawson and Tilley (1997).

A simpler form of this method is that of comparison and post-hoc matching. This approach was adopted by many early evaluations in social care (for examples, see Goldberg and Connelly, 1981). Further, this may be the only model to use if the need to evaluate arises only after the changes have been undertaken. Here, you would attempt to match the community or group that had been subject to change with another group with similar characteristics. For example, an evaluation of the Triage community care package in Connecticut was commissioned after the package was introduced, and a comparison group had to be drawn from a different area (Caro, 1981). Evaluations that use the cost–benefit analysis tool of economics are discussed in Jenkinson (1997).

Evaluation has become a more frequent element of large funded projects in recent years, as part of a trend towards accountability and measurement performance in social policy as well as other fields of public and voluntary sector work. Some government and charity schemes invite those bidding for funds to specify planned outcomes in terms of concrete results. For example, a programme to 'improve dental health' might specify that (1) the number of school pupils requiring treatment for dental caries would be reduced by say 25 per cent; (2) that 95 per cent of residents would have attended a dentist for a routine 'check-up'; and (3) that the average number of decayed teeth among primary school pupils would be halved over 3 years.

Evaluation may be controlled by a national team where there are a series of local projects (the Health Action Zones, for example) or by a locally recruited team. It is usual for the evaluators to be independent and separate from the main project. This can lead to two main sorts of difficulty. On the one hand, evaluation may start too late to see the 'before' situation and have to be rushed because of the overall schedule. On the other hand, many project leaders resent being assessed by these 'outsiders' who have a different set of values – a 'scientific' frame of reference rather than a sense of identity with the local community, for instance. Pawson and Tilley (1997) have recently argued that this can be overcome by closer collaboration at the start of a project, without the evaluators losing their objectivity.

Critics of the input/output approach to community-based evaluations argue that such research should evaluate *processes* rather than, or in addition to, outputs since

> the intervention is not sharply defined, takes different forms in different contexts and cannot be reduced to discrete components. It may not always be possible or relevant to make distinctions between cause and effect. The important questions are rather what sort of actions, in what sort of circumstances, are effective. (Curtice, 1993: 37)

Thus, many of the more recent evaluations of community-based health promotion have concentrated on the processes involved in instituting change, seeing evaluation as an on-going practice. The initial evaluation of the Drumchapel health project, for example, began during the first year of the project. This evaluation focused on specific areas of the project and investigated paid staff, volunteers and residents (McGhee and McEwen, 1993). By evaluating on-going processes, interim findings and ideas can be fed back directly into practice (see, for instance, Laughlin and Black, 1995: 145).

This processual style of evaluation is often *participative*. Thus, the Drumchapel evaluator negotiated about what and how to investigate with members of the project. In this approach evaluators play an active and collaborative role with the sponsors and main players (stakeholders). Evaluators should

> neither assume that stakeholders should act as 'respondents' providing answers to the predetermined questions of the researcher, nor assume that their task is the 'faithful' reproduction of the privileged views of the stakeholder . . . The research act thus involves 'learning' the stakeholders' theories, formalizing them, 'teaching' them back to the informant, who is then in a position to comment upon, clarify and further refine key ideas. (Pawson and Tilley, 1997: 218)

Effective community-based evaluation is thus concerned with social perspective and action, in addition to output. It should ask about

- **Numbers**   How much has been done, how many people [are] involved?
- **Processes**   What is the nature of the activities, how have people been involved?
- **Outcomes**   Has it worked? (Laughlin and Black, 1995: 142)

These questions can then be elaborated into a topic list, as for other types of research, and an appropriate method or group of methods selected.

Such processual, collaborative evaluations raise questions about information provision. In traditional evaluations outside researchers were usually commissioned to undertake investigations and report to sponsors. The project and those working on it – and those being 'acted' upon – were the subjects of the evaluation. They had no influence on the report or subsequent actions. Collaborative evaluation, on the other hand, seeks to involve all participants equally; with sponsors, project workers and public having access to the resulting information (Laughlin and Black, 1995: 141–5). This approach can, however, lead to problems, particularly in relation to control by sponsors. For example, Smithies and Adams (1993) describe how one such evaluation was halted and the report suppressed by the sponsors. Here, an Open University team was commissioned by the Health Education Authority to undertake an evaluation of community development as a method in health promotion. However, the areas investigated, staff involvement and the proposed dissemination of the report would appear to have gone beyond what the sponsors originally envisaged

> The HEA . . . did not seem to regard the participation of its staff, procedures, culture and policies as relevant topics of research . . . the intention was always that the review outcomes should be fed back to all the people that participated . . . to date the document . . . remains unpublished. (Smithies and Adams, 1993: 66–8)

The above example of things going wrong in evaluative research is not unique. Policy-related research, by definition, has a political dimension and is often, therefore, problematic. In evaluative research these problems are compounded by the number of interest groups involved (evaluated) and disagreements about ownership of the resulting knowledge.

Chapter summary

This chapter has described some of the main 'tools' and 'packages' that might be used in health needs assessments. These include the highly specialized and structured *Nottingham Health Profile, Short Form-36* and the *Townsend Disability Scale*. Other approaches described were *Priority Search*, which uses focus groups to devise question scales for larger surveys, and the *Compass* community profiling software package. *Rapid Appraisal* was also discussed.

In addition to these 'tools', researchers might make use of the *longitudinal* or *panel* approach. This method is used to collect information from the same people over time, and thus allows us to study change. However, longitudinal studies often have high drop-out rates and are very expensive. Finally, *evaluative research* was found to be particularly problematic.

Exercise

Assess the appropriateness of

1   Townsend's Disability Scale
2   the Nottingham Health Profile
3   Short Form-36
4   Rapid Appraisal
for a study of the health needs of
(a)   Older people.
(b)   A mother and toddlers' group.
(c)   A school.
(d)   A remote rural community.
(e)   An inner-urban housing estate.
(f)   Staff of a local health authority.
(g)   Women attending an ante-natal clinic.

CHAPTER 9

PROCESSING AND ANALYSIS OF QUANTITATIVE DATA

The whole purpose of collecting data is to produce *evidence* about something. In your case this is likely to be about the health needs of a particular community or group, or about comparisons between communities. Data that are collected by surveys or from existing statistical sources are *analysed* using numeric methods to produce *quantitative* evidence.

This chapter describes the procedures that might be used in this analysis. These procedures are primarily concerned with describing and summarizing the patterns and relationships of the variables in a data set using *statistical techniques*. Before this analysis can be undertaken, your raw data (questionnaires, interview schedules, official statistics etc.) have to be *processed* into a form that will allow you to analyse them.

Naturally, the way that you go about processing and analysing your data is determined by the type and amount of data that you have: the number of questionnaires, the range of topics covered and the types of questions asked. Usually, for all but the very smallest projects, you will use a computer to process and analyse your data. All of these factors influence how you will categorize the data (coding), what you look for when you analyse them (distributions, associations or predictions), and what outputs you will produce (tables, charts and graphs, for instance). The chapter is necessarily more detailed and technical than earlier ones, so it is best read more slowly, one section at a time. If you do have difficulties, seek some help.

Processing quantitative data

The first stage of processing these data is to design a *coding scheme*. You might have already done this when you designed the questionnaire, and this is recommended if at all possible. A coding scheme is a method of simplifying and standardizing the answers to each question (*variable*) into a number of categories or groups (*values*). Those giving the same answers to a particular question will be in the same group. For example, answers to a question on gender would be put in either a male group or a female group. Each question has to have all possible answers to it allocated to a particular category. If you have standardized the answers already (as 'closed questions', see Chapter 6), this is fairly straight-forward. However, if you left space for respondents to answer 'other' and to write in what that was, or if you want to group answers to open-ended questions, you will need to examine all of the answers given and attempt to devise broad categories that cover the range of responses obtained.

Clearly, for all but a small survey or range of questions, manual pro-cessing and analysis would be extremely time consuming, over complex and error prone. For a small survey it would be possible to process your data manually. In this context, a small sample might be, say, 200 cases with ten questions, or fifty cases with twenty questions. This could be done by counting, for each question, the questionnaires that have the same answers. If you wanted to compare answers for each gender or age group, you would first group your questionnaires by these categories and then further group each category by the particular answers. This is just like the counts that are made of ballot papers at a parliamentary election when the ballot papers are first sorted by candi-date before being counted. An example of this method of counting is shown in Figure 9.1.

If you have conducted a large or complex survey, you should use some form of computer processing – either using a complete package like *Compass*, a spreadsheet package (for example, Microsoft Excel, Lotus 1-2-3), or a specialist statistical package like *SPSS* (*The Statistical Package for the Social Sciences*) that allows for direct data input. This type of processing requires that you allocate a code for each answer to a question. Coding simply means translating the answers obtained into a format suitable for numeric calculations to be made. For instance, the variable 'state of health' might be coded 1 for 'very healthy', 2 for 'healthy', 3 for 'ill', 4 for 'very ill', 0 for don't know/no answer.

Although it is now usual for categories to be given numeric codes, it is not necessarily so. For instance, in the variable 'gender', females might be coded 1 or A or F and males, 2 or B or M. The main require-ment is that you are consistent: you must code all females as '1' and all males as '2', or all females as 'A' and all males as 'B', not a mixture of both. Coding may seem like a mechanical task (and, indeed, much of the final processing of questionnaires is) but the initial working out of the codes involves thinking about your data and what you want to do with them, in a rigorous way.

Information that is numeric (age, number of children, time spent in hospital etc.) can be entered as an actual value or it can be grouped. For example, you may decide to have four age groups: under 16 (coded as 1), 16–39 (coded as 2), 40–59 (coded as 3), 60 and over (coded as 4). Note

Question: State of health	Male	Female
Very healthy	* ++++ I I	* I I
Healthy	*	*
Ill	* I I I	* ++++ ++++
Very ill	*	*
Don't know/no answer	*	*

* These are 'Tally' boxes, where you keep your running totals

Figure 9.1 *Example of a manual tally*

that each category is separate with no overlap: 16–39, 40–59, not 16–40 and 40–59. It is also important to have categories for 'don't know' and 'no answer/non-response'. These are often given 0 (zero), 9 or 99 codes throughout for consistency and ease of recognition, although they can be given any code value that you do not use for any other category.

Questions that allow more than one answer (for example, Which of the following have you done in the last week?) are normally treated in one of two ways. Either you treat each answer as a question in itself (coding 1 for 'done' and 0 for 'not done') or you may decide to allow only a limited number of choices (for example, 'up to three' would be equivalent to three questions) and give each answer a unique code. The example shown in Figure 9.2 illustrates these solutions.

Once a suitable coding scheme (a 'codebook') has been designed and printed (in the *Compass* package described in Chapter 8 this would be produced automatically), each questionnaire has to be coded according to it, and the data input into the chosen computer package. Input screens usually take the form of a spreadsheet. Here each questionnaire would be a *row* and each question a *column*. It is also usual for each questionnaire to be given a unique number, as in Figure 9.3. Once the

Question:

Either   In the last week, which of the following have you done?

Or   Name **up to three** of the following things that you have done in the last week.
            Had an alcoholic drink
            Smoked tobacco
            Eaten sweets or chocolates
            Skipped a meal
            Drunk more than 5 cups of coffee in a day

Coding Scheme 1
Q Had an alcoholic drink   done = 1, not done = 0
Q Smoked tobacco   done = 1, not done = 0
Q Eaten sweets or chocolates   done = 1, not done = 0
Q Skipped a meal   done = 1, not done = 0
Q Drunk more than 5 cups of coffee   done = 1, not done = 0
  in a day

Coding Scheme 2
Q1 alcohol = 1   tobacco = 2   sweets or chocolates = 3   skipped a meal = 4   coffee = 5
Q2 alcohol = 1   tobacco = 2   sweets or chocolates = 3   skipped a meal = 4   coffee = 5
Q3 alcohol = 1   tobacco = 2   sweets or chocolates = 3   skipped a meal = 4   coffee = 5

Figure 9.2 *Example of coding multiple response questions*

information from all of the questionnaires has been entered and
checked, the data are ready to be analysed. Before this you should
ensure that you make a copy of your data set in case of damage or loss.
This copy should be kept in a different physical medium and location
to your master copy. For example, you might store the master on your
computer's hard disk at your organization and the copy on a floppy
disk at home.

Analysing quantitative data

Quantitative analysis is the way in which the processed data are
counted and statistical techniques are applied to produce descriptions
of, and associations between, the variables that form the basis of your
findings or evidence. It is important at this stage not to over analyse.
You do not necessarily need to examine the distribution of code values
for each variable. However, you should work systematically, moving
from the simple analysis of a single variable (*univariate analysis*) to the
simultaneous analysis of two (*bivariate analysis*) or more (*multivariate
analysis*) variables. If you work in this way, you will get a more thorough

| | Col 1 | Col 2 | Col 3 | Col 4 | Col 5 |
	Questionnaire Number	Question 1	Question 2	Question 3	Question 4
Row 1	0012	1	3	0	3
Row 2	0053	2	0	5	3
Row 3	0127	2	1	3	2
Row 4	etc.				
Row 5					

Figure 9.3 *Example of a spreadsheet entry*

understanding of your data, and you will be less likely to make mistakes.

It is beyond the scope of this book to describe all of the statistical techniques that you might use to analyse your data. Here, we will examine some of the most common techniques used in univariate and bivariate analysis. For more detailed descriptions of other techniques and those used in multivariate analysis, you should consult one of the many statistics textbooks that are available. Most calculations are actually carried out using computer software like *SPSS* or a spreadsheet and, provided you follow the required procedures, there is no chance of making mistakes in the arithmetic, and there is a huge time saving.

Univariate analysis

One of the first steps in data analysis is to produce *frequency counts* for the variables that we are interested in. These are simply counts of each value of the variable. For example, for the variable 'gender', we would count how many were female and how many were male. For the variable 'age group', we would count how many people were in each of the age groups that we had constructed (say, under 16; 16–29; 30–44; 45–64; 65 and over). When we first inspect our 'frequencies', we look for *outliers* or 'rogue codes': for example, if we found someone aged 302, we would expect a coding error. This error checking is part of what is called 'cleaning the data'.

Once you are happy that the counts are 'clean', they can be

Table 9.1 *Example of frequency tables*

Frequency Table 1

Gender	Number	Percentage
Male	96	48
Female	104	52
TOTAL	200	100

Frequency Table 2

State of health	Number	Percentage
Very healthy	56	28
Healthy	80	40
Ill	36	(18)
Very ill	20	(10)
Don't know/no response	8	(4)
TOTAL	200	100

Percentages in parentheses are based on small numbers.

converted into proportions or percentages to make them easier to describe: it is easier and more meaningful to say that a third or 33 per cent of our population are aged over 65 than to say that 66 of our sample of 200 are. Using proportions and percentages also makes it easier to compare variables when we come to carry out bivariate analysis.

Calculating a proportion or fraction involves dividing the count for one value by the total count. Thus, if our total sample is 250 and 100 of them are 65 and over, we would divide 100 by 250 to get two-fifths. Percentages are simply this proportion multiplied by 100: in this case 40 per cent. Although very useful, percentages and proportions are often misused by being calculated for small numbers and samples. As a general rule, if your count or your total sample is less than 50 you should not use them.

Using the two variables ('gender' and 'state of health') from Figure 9.1, we can now produce two *frequency tables*. These are shown in Table 9.1. Here we see that our sample of 200 can be divided into 96 males and 104 females, or 48 per cent and 52 per cent respectively. The frequency count for 'state of health' is more complicated than that for 'gender' because there are five possible categories (values) for this variable. Here we can also use the *mode* as a way of describing our data. The *mode* is the value that has the most cases associated with it: 'healthy' would be the *mode* in this example. Note that for the counts that are below 50 the percentages are given in parentheses.

The values for these two variables ('male', 'female' etc.) are what we

Table 9.2. *Example of an age distribution*

Raw data

Respondent number	Age in years
1	16
2	21
3	30
4	30
5	40
6	45
7	51
8	63
9	72
10	80
11	92
Total	**540**

Frequency count

Age	Count
16	1
21	1
30	2
40	1
45	1
51	1
63	1
72	1
80	1
92	1
Total	**11**

called in Chapter 3 *nominal* measurements. As we saw, we can do very little with them except simple frequency counts of the number in our sample that have each nominal value. However, if we had variables that were *interval* or *ratio* measurements, such as age, income, or height, we would be able to use their *ranges* and *means* (averages) to describe them in addition to frequency counts. A *range* is a measure of *dispersion* and a *mean* is a measure of *central tendency*. The *mode*, discussed above, and the *median* are other measures of *central tendency*.

To find out the *range* of values for a variable, you need to discover the smallest and largest values by sorting them. Table 9.2 shows the ages of a sample of eleven people listed in ascending order of age. Here the youngest person in our sample is 16 years old and the oldest person is 92 years old. The *range* is therefore 16 to 92 or '16–92'. To calculate the *mean* we first add up the ages, getting a total of 540. This is then divided by the total number in our sample (11) to give a *mean* age of 49.1 years. Only one value (30) has a count of more than one, so 30 years is the *modal* value. The *median* is the value that lies in the middle of the distribution. In this case, the sixth case (with 5 values smaller and 5 values greater) will be the *median* value: 45 years. If the sample was to comprise an even number, say 10 rather than 11, the *median* would be calculated by taking the average of the two central values. In the example they would be the fifth and sixth case – 40 plus 45 (85) divided by 2 – giving 42.5 years.

We are now in a position to describe the age distribution of our sample. We might say something like 'the ages of the people in the sample ranged from 16 to 92 years, with a mean of 49.1 years. The modal value was 30 years and the median age was 45 years'. However, it is not usual to use all of these different measures in a single description. Generally the *mean* is always calculated, and the *median* and *mode* are calculated for special cases. For example, if we wanted to know the usual or most frequent number of hours worked in a week, we would use the *mode*. Alternatively, if the mean is likely to be affected by large values at the extreme ends of the distribution, we would use the median. For instance, a couple of very elderly respondents in an otherwise young sample would make the mean much higher, and would give a poor picture of the age distribution in the sample.

In addition to the *range*, we can use a measure called the *variance* to

Table 9.3 *Calculation of variance and standard deviation*

Respondent number	Age in years	Deviation from mean	Deviation squared
1	16	−133.1	1095.61
2	21	−28.1	789.61
3	30	−19.1	364.81
4	30	−19.1	364.81
5	40	−9.1	82.81
6	45	−4.1	16.81
7	51	1.9	3.61
8	63	13.9	193.21
9	72	22.9	524.41
10	80	30.9	954.81
11	92	42.9	1840.41
Total	**540**	**0**	**6230.91**

Variance	**6230.91/10**
	= 623.1
Standard Deviation	$\sqrt{623.1}$
	= 24.96

get an estimate of the variability or scatter of the values of a variable: how they vary from the *mean* value. This is calculated by first measuring the difference (or *deviation*) that each recorded value is from the *mean* value. If these differences were added, the total would always be zero: the negative and positive differences from the *mean* would cancel each other out. Instead, the differences are squared, totalled and divided by the sample size minus 1. The resulting number is called the *variance*. The calculation of the *variance* of our age variable is shown in Table 9.3.

Associated with this is what is termed the *standard deviation* (the average deviation from the sample mean). This is derived by calculating the square root of the *variance*. *Standard deviations* are high when the values are widely scattered (as in the age variable in Table 9.3) and low when they are close to the *mean*. *Standard deviation* is an important concept in significance tests, discussed later in this chapter.

The *standard deviation* is also used to *normalize* variables as an aid to comparison in bivariate and multivariate analysis. For example, if you wanted to compare variables that used different scales of measurement (for instance, unemployment and morbidity, or where examination marks are based on different scoring systems), you might first of all *normalize* the values of each variable and then compare the resulting values. The most frequently used method is called the *z-transformation*. Here, the raw values are converted into *z-scores* by first subtracting the *mean* value from the recorded value and then dividing by the *standard deviation*. Each variable will now have a *mean* of zero and a *standard deviation* of 1, and the variables can be compared more easily. Thus, in Table 9.3, the fifth person would have a *z-score* for age of (40 − 49.1) divided by 24.96, giving −0.36. These could be used instead of the actual value in other computations. For example, they are used in the construction of the *Townsend Material Deprivation Index*, discussed in Chapter 4.

Bivariate analysis

Usually, we do not want to produce evidence that is simply based on the descriptions of single variables. We want to look at relationships between variables: for example, the relationship between health status and occupation or, at the area level, morbidity and deprivation. To do this we have to make comparisons and associations. The types of statistical techniques that we use to investigate these relationships are determined by the level of measurement of the variables: nominal, ordinal, interval or ratio.

The first step in this process is the production of a cross-tabulation or *contingency table*. These tables are in the form of grids that have one variable and its values listed across the rows of the grid and the other variable and its values listed down the columns. When we read across a row to where it intersects with the column, we find the number of cases that have the value for that row and that column. Each intersecting 'box' is called a *cell* in a contingency table. It is usual for the dependant variable (the one that is affected) to be listed in the rows and the independent variable (the one that might bring about the effect) listed in the columns. Sometimes it might not be clear which is dependent. In such cases you would use a common sense approach and list the variable with the fewest values in the columns. The first part of Table 9.4 ('Full Count') shows a typical contingency table for the two variables 'gender' and 'state of health', used in the previous discussion.

Here we see that a count is made for each combination of variable values and recorded in the appropriate cell, so that we have, for instance, 32 males who are 'very healthy' and 20 females who are 'ill'. These tables also show totals for each row and column (called *marginal totals* or just *marginals*) and a grand total in the bottom right-hand corner. If you construct these tables manually, a good way of checking for arithmetic

Table 9.4 *Example of contingency tables*

Full count

Health status	Gender		
	Male	Female	**Total**
Very healthy	32 (33)	24 (23)	**56 (28)**
Healthy	40 (42)	40 (38)	**80 (40)**
III	16 (17)	20 (19)	**36 (18)**
Very ill	8 (8)	12 (12)	**20 (10)**
Don't know/No response	0 (0)	8 (8)	**8 (4)**
Total	**96 (100)**	**104 (100)**	**200 (100)**

Excluding non-response

Health status	Gender		
	Male	Female	**Total**
Very healthy	32 (33)	24 (29)	**56 (29)**
Healthy	40 (42)	40 (42)	**80 (42)**
III	16 (17)	20 (21)	**36 (19)**
Very ill	8 (8)	12 (13)	**20 (10)**
Total	**96 (100)**	**96 (100)**	**192 (100)**

Column percentages shown in parentheses are rounded to the nearest whole number.

or tally errors is by checking the marginal totals. On visual inspection we see that there are slight differences in health status between males and females, with 33 per cent of males being 'very healthy' and only 8 per cent 'very ill', compared with female rates of 23 per cent and 12 per cent respectively. However, 8 of our female respondents gave no categorical answer to the question and should be ignored in this analysis. The resulting table is shown in the second part of Table 9.4.

We now need to find out if there is a relationship between gender and health status: are the differences between 33 per cent and 29 per cent, and/or between 8 per cent and 13 per cent really (*significantly*) different, or could they have occurred by chance as a result of sampling errors. When there are large differences in the proportions (say there were 50 per cent 'very healthy' males and 2 per cent 'very healthy' females), it is highly likely that a relationship does exist. However, in the majority of cases it is necessary to do a *significance test*. These are described later in this chapter.

Table 9.5A *Raw data for health status score*

Case number	Age	Health score
1	16	92
2	21	80
3	30	75
4	30	80
5	40	75
6	45	62
7	51	64
8	63	30
9	72	44
10	80	35
11	92	40

Table 9.5B *A grouped contingency table for interval level data*

| Health score | Age group | | | | |
	16–26	30–44	45–64	65+	Total
0–40	0	0	1	3	4
50–79	0	2	2	0	4
80+	2	1	0	0	3
Total	**2**	**3**	**3**	**3**	**11**

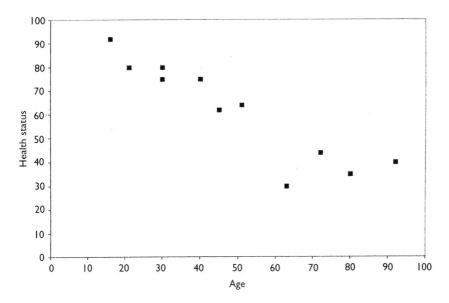

Figure 9.4 *Example of a scatter plot*

When the values of our variables are of ordinal, interval or ratio levels of measurement, we might find that the number of cells that resulted made it impossible to interpret. In this case we could group the values. For example, our sample of eleven people of various ages each have a health status score that ranges from 30 to 92 (Table 9.5A). So that we might visually examine the relationship between age and health status, we could combine values of each variable into the groupings shown in Table 9.5B. Here, instead of the 10-by-9 table (with 90 cells) that we would have produced had we used the raw values, our data have been reduced to a 3-by-4 table (with 12 cells), making interpretation much easier. On visual inspection of Table 9.5B there appears to be a fairly clear relationship between age and health status. Those in the older age group all have low health status scores and those in the younger age group have high health status scores.

This relationship could also be examined visually by constructing a *scatter plot* graph from the raw data. This is shown in Figure 9.4. Here we see the intersecting scores forming a fairly straight line sloping down to the right. This slope suggests a strong 'negative' relationship. Had it sloped down to the left, the relationship would be said to be 'positive'. A negative relationship is one in which the values of one variable increase as the values of the other decrease – they move in opposite directions. A positive relationship is one where the values both increase or both decrease – they move in the same direction.

Associations and causes

Up to this point, we have been careful to talk about the possible *relation-ship* between variables, because we wanted to use common sense terms. In quantitative analysis it is more usual to use the word *association* as a general word that covers all types of effects between variables. As it is a general word, it does not imply that any one variable is independent or dependent, or that one *causes* another. It is a very strong statement to say that one thing is 'caused' by another. Strictly speaking, our evidence normally shows that the values of one variable tend to be associated with (happen with, in our sample) certain values of another variable. Research results are seldom that neat.

A far more typical finding is that 'more people in this group are likely to experience something, than do the people in that group'. In Table 9.4 we saw that more women than men are likely to say that they are 'ill' or 'very ill'. However, we cannot say gender 'causes' reported ill health, because Table 9.4 also shows us that most women are healthy, and some men also say they are ill. The best we can say is that women are more prone to (have a higher *probability* of reporting that they have) ill health. That is why social researchers rarely use the word 'cause'.

In much the same way, in everyday language people say that there is a 'correlation' between two things. When we are talking in social research language, the term *correlation* has a specific meaning, based on a statistical technique. This is best thought of by visualizing a scatter plot similar to the one shown in Figure 9.4, with a straight line drawn through the points on the graph in such a way that the line best represents the pattern. If the points are close to the line, the two variables are *correlated*, if they are widely scattered, they are not.

The most commonly used correlation technique is called *Pearson's product-moment correlation coefficient* or 'r'. This is usually calculated using a computer but will be worked out manually here for demonstration purposes. The correlation coefficient is calculated by using the formula

$$r = \frac{N\Sigma xy - (\Sigma x)(\Sigma y)}{\sqrt{[N\Sigma x^2 - (\Sigma x)^2][N\Sigma y^2 - (\Sigma y)^2]}}$$

where N is the number in the sample; Σ is the summation sign; x is the value of one variable; y is the value of the other variable, and $\sqrt{}$ is the square root symbol. The coefficient r is always in the range –1 to +1. The closer the coefficient is to 1 or –1, the stronger the association. When r is 0 (zero) there is no association. Negative values represent a negative correlation and positive values represent a positive correlation between the variables. The manual calculations for our health status and age example are shown in Table 9.6.

Table 9.6 *Calculation of Pearson's product moment correlation coefficient (r)*

Age (x)	Health status (y)	xy	x^2	y^2
16	92	1472	256	8464
21	80	1680	441	6400
30	75	2250	900	5625
30	80	2400	900	6400
40	75	3000	1600	5625
45	62	2790	2025	3844
51	64	3264	2601	4096
63	30	1890	3969	900
72	44	3168	5184	1936
80	35	2800	6400	1225
92	40	3680	8464	1600
Σ 540	677	28394	32740	46115

Applying the formula

$$r = \frac{[11 \times (28394)] - [(540) \times (677)]}{\sqrt{[(11 \times 32740) - (540)^2] \times [(11 \times 46115) - (677)^2]}}$$

$$= \frac{-53246}{57914.36}$$

$$= -0.9194$$

Note: usually the multiplication sign '×' or '*' is omitted so that ( )( ) means multiply the number in the first set of parentheses by the number in the second set.

Here we find that the correlation coefficient is –0.9194, which suggests a strong negative association between age and health status in our sample. The square of the coefficient, r^2, is a measure of the amount of *variance* in the distribution that can be explained by the two variables. In this case 0.85 or 85 per cent of the variability can be explained by age and health status, and only 15 per cent (100 per cent minus 85 per cent) is the result of chance.

It must be stressed again that correlation is a method of assessing the *association* or relationship between variables. It does not suggest *causality* nor does it allow predictions to be made. Predictions are made by using the *regression technique*. This technique is used to calculate a straight line through a scatter plot, like the one shown in Figure 9.4. Methods of calculating regression lines are described in most statistics textbooks.

Often data are expressed in terms of ranks (*ordinal*) rather than in intervals. In such cases, *Spearman's rank-order correlation coefficient*, 'r_s', may be calculated. This calculation uses the differences in the rankings achieved on two variables. Other techniques that might be used for ordinal data include *Tau, Gamma* and *Sommer's D*. Full details of these formulae are given in all major statistics textbooks.

One of the main problems we meet when using correlation and regression is that the standard methods only work for a relationship that is linear, as in Figure 9.4. If instead of a straight line our data showed a curve, the results of the correlation would suggest a weak association. For example, if our first three respondents had health status scores of 45, 45 and 50 (because they were unfit or physically disabled, for instance), the resulting r would be -0.45, and the r^2 would be 0.2. We might therefore interpret this as implying a very weak relationship, even though there was really an underlying association. Such curvilinear relationships are best identified by inspection of the scatter plots, and tests for *non-linearity* could then be undertaken. If you suspect this pattern in your data, it is advisable to consult a statistician since tests for non-linearity are very difficult.

Significance tests

When you take a *random* sample, your aim is to obtain a sample that is representative of your chosen population. You can then make generalizations about the base population from the findings of your particular sample. However, because your evidence is only derived from a sample of your population, you cannot be sure that the results obtained have arisen by chance. You therefore need some way of calculating how good an estimate your findings are of those that would have been obtained from your population as a whole. In addition, you need a way of assessing the strength of the relationships that you have found. *Significance tests* are used to answer these questions.

Many different tests have been developed for the various levels of measurement and for the various types of analysis. Some of these are based on the assumption that the frequency distributions of the variables in the population have a particular pattern, called a *Gaussian* or 'normal' distribution. This distribution is a symmetrical bell-shaped curve, with the *mean* value of the variable at the centre and highest point of the curve. Examples of this distribution are shown in practically all statistical texts. The most important feature of this distribution, for our purposes, is that 68 per cent of the population would have a value for the variable of the mean plus or minus 1 standard deviation; plus or minus 1.6 standard deviations would cover 90 per cent of the population; plus or minus 2 standard deviations would cover 95 per cent; and 99 per cent of the population would fall between the mean and 2.6 standard deviations. Significance tests based on this distribution (called *parametric* tests) use this feature to determine *significance* or *probability levels* (*p*) – 90 per cent or .1; 95 per cent or .05; and 99 per cent or .01. This distribution is not 'normal' in the sense of being 'usual' or 'generally the case', rather it is the distribution that much of statistical theory is based upon. Significance tests not based upon this distribution are called *non-parametric*. However, they also use the same significance levels.

The first step in carrying out a significance test is to set up a *null hypothesis* (often referred to as 'H_0'). This is usually of the form that 'there is no relationship between variables *x* and *y*' or 'the findings are not significant'. A significance test is then carried out to test this. The results obtained are then compared with values that have been previously calculated by statisticians. The null hypothesis can then be 'rejected' or 'accepted'.

For nominal level data, the most widely used significance test is the non-parametric chi-square (χ^2) test or 'goodness of fit' test. 'χ^2' is pronounced 'Ki-squared'. This test can be used for univariate, bivariate and multivariate analysis. Other significance tests for this level of measurement include *Fisher's exact test*, the *z-test of proportions*, *McNemar* and *Cochran Q*. The χ^2 test compares the observed frequencies with those expected from the marginal totals. For example, in the first part of Table 9.7 (on p. 138), to ease manual computation, the contingency table shown in Table 9.5B has been regrouped into a 2-by-2 table: male and female by 'healthy' and 'ill'. Our null hypothesis is that there is no relationship between gender and health status, and we will select the 95 per cent probability level (.05 level).

The formula for χ^2 is $\chi^2 = \Sigma(o - e)^2/e$, where *o* is the observed frequency and *e* is the expected frequency. The expected frequency is calculated by taking the proportion of the total of one set of marginals and applying this to the other marginal. In our example, 136 divided by 192 gives a proportion of 0.71, and 56 divided by 192 gives 0.29. In the lower part of Table 9.7 these proportions are applied to the column marginal totals to give the expected frequencies. Each of these are then subtracted from the equivalent observed frequency, the result is then squared and divided by the expected frequency. These are then added together to give 3.76. We then have to compare this result with a table of the χ^2 distribution. These tables are found in most statistics textbooks.

Because χ^2 can be used for tables containing any number of rows and columns, the χ^2 distribution shows values at different significance levels for what are called *degrees of freedom*. *Degrees of freedom* refers to the number of cells that are needed to be known before it is possible to work out the others from the marginal totals. They are calculated by subtracting 1 from the number of columns and multiplying this by the number of rows minus 1. In our example a 2-by-2 table would have (2 – 1) multiplied by (2 – 1) or 1 degree of freedom. If it had been a 6-by-3 table, the degrees of freedom would have been $(6 - 1)$ multiplied by $(3 - 1)$ or 10. Using the χ^2 distribution table for our worked example, the value of χ^2 at 1 degree of freedom and a probability level of .05 would have to be 3.84 or more before we could reject the null hypothesis. Our result of 3.76 is lower than this, and we must therefore accept the null hypothesis that there is no relationship between gender and health status.

If we had used a probability level of .1, the value of χ^2 to reject the null hypothesis would be 2.71, and in our case we could reject it at this level, and accept that there is a relationship between gender and health status. The choice of probability or significance level is determined by the researcher. Usually, the .05 (or 95 per cent) level is selected. However, if one wanted to be more certain that the findings had not occurred by chance, the .01 (99 per cent) level could be selected. Alternatively, if you were satisfied with a 90 per cent chance of being correct, you could use the .1 level.

Non-parametric significance tests for levels of measurement above the nominal level include the *Kolmogorov–Smirnov test, Mann–Whitney U-test*, the *runs test*, the *sign test* and the *Wilcoxon test* for ordinal data. For interval and ratio level data, the most frequent tests are the parametric t, z and F tests. These are all described in standard statistics textbooks.

To test the significance of our correlation results in Table 9.6, we could use a distribution table for *rho*, similar to the χ^2 distribution. However, this can only be used for sample sizes of 30 or less. For a larger sample the *t-statistic* is used. In our example, the results are significant at the .01 level; with r being greater than the 0.746 value needed for a sample of this size.

Multivariate techniques

Because quantitative analysis ranges from the straightforward, like percentages or means, to the more complicated, like significance tests, this chapter has moved in progressive stages, starting with univariate methods and then moving on to bivariate techniques. It will not have escaped the reader's notice that while some matters can be dealt with at these levels, in real life most issues involve more than one or two variables. To return to the earlier example, the greater illness reported among the women in our sample might be something to do with their age, rather than their gender. In this situation, we have three variables instead of two. Our example is now more like ordinary life.

To express this in research terms, close associations between variables might occur, not because the two variables are directly related, but because a third, *intervening variable* is associated with both. This apparent association between two variables is called a *spurious* relationship. The usual way of testing for this is to carry out the test of association with the intervening variable *held constant*. Holding a variable constant means that we look at the relationship between the other two for each separate value of the variable held constant. When we calculate the resulting coefficient, and find that it is very low, it is probable that the original relationship was spurious.

In our example, we need to discover if gender is associated with illness in the same way among young, middle aged and older respondents. This can sometimes be easily checked by splitting up the original table into several tables, one for each of the values of the variable held constant. If the data are not too complex, a contingency table can then be reconstructed showing two variables on one axis, and one on the other axis. You can have even more variables presented in this way, but reading and understanding the outcome gets progressively more difficult.

It is important that you never assume that, because two variables are associated, one is creating the effect in the other. You should always ask yourself if another, as yet unconsidered or unknown, variable is *intervening*. A number of sophisticated statistical techniques exist for this, and offer interesting ways of mapping complex associations and reducing complicated patterns to a more simple summary. Although inexperienced researchers should be cautioned against using these, it is worth knowing some of their names (such *as multiple regression, path analysis, factor analysis, cluster analysis, log-linear modelling*) so that they can be recognized if they are encountered in the literature. The only sensible thing to do, whether you are bewildered by them or tempted to use them, is to seek help from somebody who does understand them properly.

Epidemiological analysis

A full discussion of the techniques used in epidemiology is beyond the scope of this book, and those wishing to use these methods should refer to any of the many textbooks on this subject. However, when using secondary data, you are likely to come across various measurements used by epidemiologists. These include *incidence* and *prevalence* rates, *mortality* and *birth* rates, and *standardizations*. The most common ones are therefore described here.

Measurements of the distribution of disease in a population are often given in terms of rates per thousand, ten thousand or even per hundred thousand of the *population at risk*. This is to make the measurements meaningful and to allow for comparisons to be made. For example, that there were ten cases of lung cancer in a community means very little unless we know what proportion of the population this represents, and whether it is worse or better than the national figure.

The most common rates that are used in epidemiology are *incidence* and *prevalence*. These are often confused. The *incidence* of a disease refers to the rate at which *new cases* of the disease occur in a population during a specified time period. Thus you will find incidence rates expressed as 10 new cases per 100,000 per year or 6 new cases per 1,000 per year, or whatever time period is selected. *Prevalence*, on the other hand, refers to the *total number of cases* in a specified period. For example, we might say that in a population of 10,000 males over 16 years of age, 50 new cases of lung cancer occurred last year. The total number of cases of lung cancer in that period was 250. The first figure (50) would be used to express the *incidence*, and the second figure (250) would be used to express the *prevalence*.

The various birth and fertility rates also cause confusion. A crude *birth rate* is the number of live births expressed as a proportion of the mid-year estimates of the population. These mid-year estimates are produced every year by the Office for National Statistics and published in *Population Trends*. They are, as the term suggests, the best estimate that can be made of the size of the population for a particular year. The *fertility rate* uses the more sophisticated denominator of women between the ages of 15 and 44 (the 'at risk' population). Another rate relating to births is the *Infant Mortality Rate*, which can be defined as the number of infant deaths (under one year) in a year expressed as a proportion of the number of live births occurring in that year.

Many different *mortality rates* are calculated. These include the crude death rate and disease and age/gender specific rates. One of the most useful of the specific rates is the *Standard Mortality Ratio* or *SMR*. This ratio is used when comparisons need to be made. For example, if crude death rates were used to compare areas in the UK, places such as Torquay or Christchurch would have much higher rates than Swindon or Luton. This is not because the people of Swindon and Luton are more healthy than those of Torquay or Christchurch, rather these latter two places have a much higher number of older people (who are more likely to die) in their population.

To get around this problem, first, the death rates are calculated for each gender and age group in the total population (of the UK or England and Wales, for instance). These rates are then applied to the numbers in each age and gender group in the sub-population to obtain estimates of the expected number of deaths. The estimates are then added to give an overall estimate of the deaths that would occur in a particular sub-population with a given age and gender distribution. This estimate is then used with the actual (observed) number of deaths to calculate the SMR. The formula used is $o/e * 100$ – the observed number (*o*) divided by (/) the expected number (*e*), multiplied by (*) 100. This ensures that the SMR for the total population is always 100. An SMR that is below 100 shows a lower than average death rate, and an SMR of over 100 shows a higher than expected one. These and other terms are described in the Glossary.

Graphic outputs

In addition to producing tabulation, coefficients and rates from your data, it is often more understandable to construct graphs and charts. These can make the identification of patterns easier than from an inspection of a table of numbers. For example, the *scatter plot* shown in Figure 9.4 shows the relationship between age and health status much more clearly than does the frequency distribution in Table 9.5.

The most popular graphical representations are *bar charts*, *pie charts* and *graphs*. Many different types of these can now be easily produced using a computer spreadsheet package such as Excel. Bar charts or *histograms* show the counts of the different values of a variable as blocks of varying size, while in pie charts these are shown as proportions or

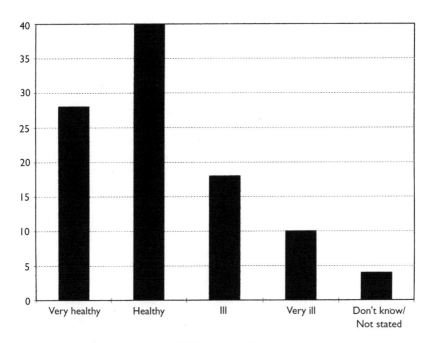

Figure 9.5 *Example of a bar chart*

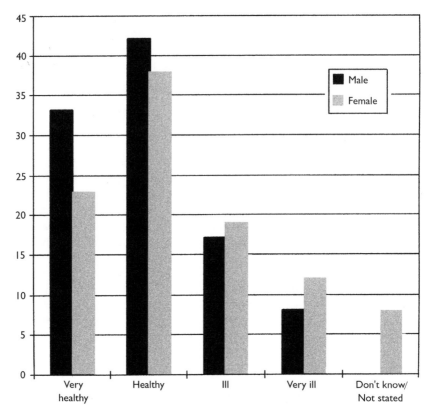

Figure 9.6 *Example of a two variable bar chart*

slices. Examples of bar and pie charts, using data from the gender and health status example, are given in Figures 9.5–9.7. Graphs should only be used for interval or ratio data that vary over time. Here the values are joined in a continuous line. An example of a graph is given in Figure 9.8.

Chapter summary

This chapter has been longer, more detailed and technical than earlier ones because of the many statistical methods and terms that it has covered. However, if you are going to undertake a survey or analyse existing statistical data, it is important that you understand the most widely used techniques, even if you use a computer for your data processing.

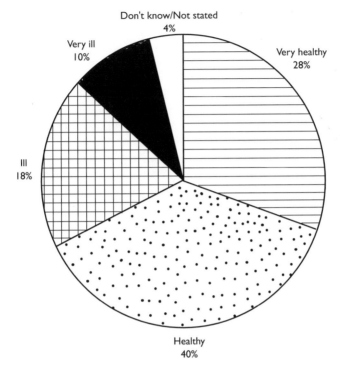

Figure 9.7 *Example of a pie chart*

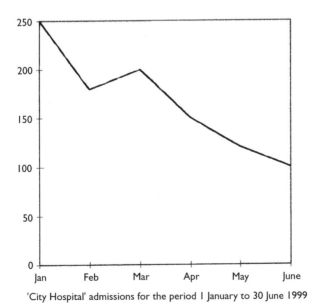

'City Hospital' admissions for the period 1 January to 30 June 1999

Figure 9.8 *Example of a graph*

We started the chapter by looking at ways of describing single variables (*univariate analysis*), and then moved through methods of examining relationships between two variables (*bivariate analysis*) to *multivariate* approaches. In addition, *significance tests*, the most common *epidemiological techniques* and *graphical outputs* were discussed.

Single variables are usually described in terms of measures of *central tendency* (*mean*, *median* and *mode*) and their *range* of values (*frequency counts or tables*). The range or spread of interval or ratio measured variables can also be described using *variance* and *standard deviation*. Bivariate analysis, on the other hand, looks at *associations* between variables using *contingency tables*, *correlation* and *regression*. When we use *multivariate* techniques, we begin to examine more complex data relationships. These should only be undertaken by those competent in advanced statistics.

Table 9.7 *A worked example of the χ^2 test*

Observed

	Male	Female	**Total**
Healthy	72	64	136
Ill	24	32	56
Total	**96**	**96**	**192**

Computation

o	e	o − e	$(o - e)^2$	$(o - e)^2/e$
72	68	4	16	0.24
64	68	−4	16	0.24
24	28	−4	16	0.57
32	28	4	16	0.57
				$\chi^2 = 3.76$

Exercise

In Table 9.8 the Townsend Material Deprivation Index and the Jarman UPA score are given for 20 areas. Using *Pearson's product moment correlation coefficient*, describe the relationship between these two deprivation measures.

Table 9.8 *Deprivation scores for the exercise*

Ward number	Townsend index	UPA score
1	5.18	23.08
2	−0.29	−2.20
3	2.78	16.50
4	2.31	13.31
5	−0.64	−8.53
6	−0.49	−2.84
7	5.26	24.61
8	3.73	18.45
9	5.05	29.31
10	3.53	15.99
11	−2.66	−3.83
12	−3.41	−13.30
13	−2.58	−11.41
14	−0.92	−2.84
15	4.13	22.88
16	9.41	48.77
17	2.12	3.17
18	3.21	16.85
19	6.11	30.63
20	0.42	4.82

CHAPTER 10

PROCESSING AND ANALYSIS OF QUALITATIVE DATA

Unlike quantitative data, the information collected for qualitative analysis does not come in a standardized format on a questionnaire, interview schedule or in a statistical table. Instead, it may be in the form of notes, audio tapes, diaries, documents, newspapers, visual images or a mixture of these. The objective of processing and analysing these qualitative data is to transform them to text and, as with quantitative processing, to categorize and code the text so that it may be interpreted to produce evidence and understanding.

These procedures are, however, less well defined, documented or neatly prescribed than quantitative methods. Not least, analysis does not wait for the end of the data collection before it all takes place in a single phase. Thus, we saw in Chapter 7, that analysis might be undertaken during the collection stage in the form of *theoretical sampling*. Further, qualitative analysis is often an iterative process that involves the increasing refinement of concepts and the testing and re-testing of interpretations. Despite these features, it is possible, for our purposes, to divide the procedures involved into four distinct tasks: transcription; preliminary data inspection; content analysis; interpretation.

In addition to these four processes, this chapter describes methods of interpreting visual data. Although not common in health research, the analysis of visual data can offer important insights for community needs assessment. Finally, methods of computer-assisted qualitative analysis are considered.

Qualitative methods cannot be regarded as a unified set of research procedures. The particular methodological approach that is adopted is very much determined by the theoretical and paradigmatic perspective of the researcher. The competing approaches to qualitative research include ethnography, grounded theory, phenomenology, action research, postmodernist and feminist research. In this chapter, the main features of what might be called 'mainstream-traditional' qualitative analysis will be described. These are likely to be the most useful for the projects that you might be involved in. Those wishing to examine the alternative approaches should consult texts such as Grbich (1999), Sarantakos (1993) and Silverman (1993).

From data to text

If we are dealing with one or two very short and straightforward examples of qualitative data (a brief conversation, some notes of a conversation, or some very preliminary and early event in the research process, for instance) we might analyse it in a common sense way. This might mean reading it through a few times, and thinking where it might lead us in the research. But *systematic qualitative research* has to be far more thorough, and is very hard work.

The first task in the processing of qualitative data is to get the information into a format suitable for classifying and ordering. If possible, all hand-written field notes, interview notes and diaries should be typed up – preferably using a word processing package – to make them easy to read. If this is not possible, they should at least be made legible. This should be undertaken as soon as possible after the information has been collected. Quickly made notes that appear understandable at the time are often difficult to make sense of afterwards. It is surprising how frequently valuable data are lost because of this. It is also important to ensure that the date, the name of the person who made the notes – or a cross-referenced code if it is a respondent – and other relevant background details are recorded. If a word processing package is used, this information could be entered in the 'header' or 'footer' section.

Newspaper articles and other documents should also be transferred to a standard format if possible. If these are too long to transcribe, they could be photocopied onto A4 sheets, and a note could be made of the source details on these. Alternatively, if you have access to a scanner with optical character recognition (OCR) software, these documents could be scanned in and translated into the same computer file format as your other transcriptions. When photocopying or scanning, always try to leave a large left-hand margin for adding your notes later.

When information is in the form of audio tapes, it will have to be transcribed into written format. This usually involves verbatim transcription, and should not be cleaned up. Sometimes this happens when the transcriber wants to 'correct the English' or take out all those 'mmms'. This process takes a considerable amount of time and patience. As a rule of thumb, transcription time will be between three and five times the length of the original recording. Sometimes it may be impossible to transcribe all audio recordings verbatim. In this case, detailed notes should be made, and the corresponding tape-counter readings should be noted against each separate theme.

Transcriptions and note-taking are especially difficult if respondents have unusual accents, are soft spoken or when there is more than one respondent: in group discussions for example. Group discussions are particularly problematic because of the difficulties in identifying individual speakers. In such cases, hopefully, notes or codes to their identity will have been made during the discussion. As with written documents and notes, details of the date, time, respondent code and other relevant information should be recorded with each transcription and a wide left-hand margin provided on the text pages.

Ideally, this initial process will have produced a set of 'texts' that can be stored and retrieved both electronically and manually: in a computer *and* in your filing cabinet – and *always* have more than one copy. These could be organized by the type of text (interview, notes, diaries, for instance) and by any other organizing principle that is thought relevant. These texts are then ready for data analysis.

Preliminary data inspection

The first stage in the analysis of qualitative data involves reading through the text of each interview, observation or other type of document to get an overall impression of the data. Here each account is read as a whole. This involves summarizing the text, making notes in the margin, adding reflexive accounts, and identifying significant words, phrases or passages that might be used in the more detailed analysis or for illustrative quotations. While doing this, the text is cleaned up (checked for transcription errors and omissions, irrelevancies etc.) and sorted into broad groups.

These groupings will be determined by the original aims of the research. For example, groupings could be by age, gender, occupation, household size, household stage or type, or health status. Each text is then cross-referenced according to the selected groupings. Some form of symbol or colour coding could be used on the front of each text to ease subsequent identification. It is also usual to create an index that lists text references for each grouping. This could be done by using index cards or by creating separate computer files. Figure 10.1 shows how this might be done. Any separate summaries are either attached to the main text or, more usually, the text's reference code is indicated on the summary sheet itself.

An example of the type of analysis that is undertaken during this preliminary stage is given in Figure 10.2. In the first box a diary entry from Townsend's 1950s study of older people is given as it appears in his report (Townsend, 1963: 296–7), but with my highlighting and marginal notes. In the second box is my initial interpretation, based on these notes. Here, attention is drawn to the routine domestic chores, meal patterns and content, family, neighbours and friends, and leisure. The original instructions given to the diarists were 'to note the time of day when

Interview text   **Index cards**

Reference number:	034
Age group:	24–39
Household size:	3
Occupation:	Prof & Tech (b)
Gender:	F

Transcript of interview ~~~~~

Age Group: 24–39

012

023

034

048

Household size: 3

006

010

034

050

Occupation: Prof & Tech (b)

001

033

034

036

Gender: F

002

003

012

034

Figure 10.1 *Example of cross referencing in qualitative analysis*

	Mrs Tucker, 16 Bantam Street, aged *sixty*, living with *infirm* husband in *terraced cottage*	Line No.
	Monday	
order of chores	7.45 a.m. I got up, went down, and put *my* kettle on the gas – half-way – then I	1
	raked *my* fire out and laid it, swept *my* ashes up, and then cleaned *my* hearth.	2
	Then I set light to *my* fire, then sat down for a while, then I made *tea* and *me and*	3
naming	*Dad* had a cup.	4
shopping	9.20 a.m. I went out for the *Daily Mirror* and *fags for Dad*. About eight people said	5
people/neighbours	'Good Morning' with a nice smile, then I replied back. Then I went home and	6
	prepared oats and bread, butter and tea and me and *Dad* sat for *breakfast*. When	7
chores	we finished *I cleared away and swept and mopped my kitchen out.*	8
cooking	11.15 a.m. I started to *get dinner on*, then Mrs Rice, *a neighbour*, asked me to get	9
neighbour/	her *coals in*, and *she will take my bag-wash*, also get *my dog's meat*. We had a	10
reciprocity/chat	nice chat about *Mother's Day*. I showed her my flowers and card which Alice	11
[	sent. It was very touching, a box of chocs from John, stockings and card from	12
family[	Rose, card and 5s. from Bill, as I know they all think dearly of me.	13
visit from/meal-food	1.0 p.m. *My daughter Alice came with baby*. We had *dinner together.*	14
visit from/drink-snack	2.0 p.m. *My daughter Rose and husband* came. I made *a cup of tea and cake.*	15
leisure	3.15 p.m. *Dad* and I sat to *listen to radio.*	16
meal	5.0 p.m. We both had *tea, bread and cheese Dad, bread and jam myself.* When	17
chores	finished *I cleared away again.*	18
visit from/check -	7.0 p.m. *My son John and his wife* called to see *if we were all right* before they went	19
concern	home from *work.*	20
chores	8.0 p.m. I did *a little mending.*	21
	10.0 p.m. We *went to bed.*	22

Summary

Female, married, 60. Sick partner.

Routine **domestic chores** – orderly routine on getting up: got up, went downstairs, put kettle on, raked fire out, laid fire, swept ashes, cleaned hearth, lit fire, made tea, shopping, made breakfast, cleared up, cleaned kitchen, prepared dinner, made tea, cleared up after tea, did some mending. Refers to 'my' kettle, 'my' fire, 'my' kitchen, etc.
Division of labour – appears to do everything – husband 'infirm'.
Food/meals – these punctuate the day. Early morning tea, breakfast after paper – ?for spouse to read?, dinner (main meal at mid-day), tea and cakes for p.m. family visitors, their tea (light meal – bread + other – spouse, cheese, she, jam ?cost – man gets the protein?). No mention of any drinks or meal after this.
Family – spouse, 2 daughters, 2 sons, son-in-law, daughter-in-law, grandchild. Refers to husband as 'Dad'. Children referred to by first names, others by relationship to them. Children visited – given meals/tea – Mother's Day, so all offspring visit. Presents and cards. **'they all think dearly of me'**. Son and wife check to see if they're all right – no mention of this checking by other offspring.
Neighbours/friends – met 8 people she knew while shopping, exchanged pleasantries. Chat with neighbour – called for favour – reciprocity. Talked about MD and family.
Leisure – occasional sit down. Listening to radio. ?dog.

Figure 10.2 *Example of preliminary data inspection (original text from Townsend, 1963: 296–7, with highlighting (italic) added)*

getting up, having breakfast, calling on relations and friends, etc.'. These have clearly influenced the categories identified in the summary.

As this is only an illustration, the preliminary analysis has only been carried out on a single diary entry for one person. Normally it would be undertaken for all diary entries and an overall summary would then be made. This analysis would be undertaken for each diary. The diaries for each respondent could then be sorted into relevant groupings and suitably indexed.

Clearly, the large amount of text that is generated by qualitative methods means that any analysis would be severely limited unless a suitable filing system is established. As discussed above, texts, summaries and indexes can be stored as computer 'files' for predominantly computer analysis. However, these should be organized and labelled so that identification and access is straightforward, in separate computer 'folders' for example. Further, the amount of manual sifting, sorting and marking that is carried out during this data inspection phase means that a suitable manual filing system is imperative. Here, each different type of text could be stored, alphabetically or in reference number order, in a separate drawer or box file. Index cards could be used for each category, and again filed in alphabetic or numeric order. It is also important to remember that all the notes and summaries that are made during analysis should be treated as text, and suitably stored.

Content analysis

Once the preliminary sorting and categorizing of all the texts has been carried out, it is probable that some broad themes will have been identified. The next stage is the identification and classification of all possible categories and concepts that are found in the texts. This involves going through the texts again, looking for words and phrases that describe a process, concept, relationship or category. This process might be seen as devising a coding scheme for the data, with the identified words and phrases indicating possible variables.

Each word, phrase, concept and category is noted down along with the text reference number and the page, paragraph and line number within the text. It is also common, particularly with newspaper and documentary analysis, to measure the number of column inches or count the lines that are devoted to each category in each text. A content analysis of the first part of the diary text in Table 10.1 might result in the following items

Got up: Respondent number 001/Diary/Day 1/Line 1
Went down: Respondent number 001/Diary/Day 1/Line 1
Kettle on: Respondent number 001/Diary/Day 1/Line 1
Raked fire: Respondent number 001/Diary/Day 1/Line 2
Laid fire: Respondent number 001/Diary/Day 1/Line 2
Swept ashes: Respondent number 001/Diary/Day 1/Line 2
Cleaned hearth: Respondent number 001/Diary/Day 1/Line 2
Lit fire: Respondent number 001/Diary/Day 1/Line 3
Sat down: Respondent number 001/Diary/Day 1/Line 3
Made tea: Respondent number 001/Diary/Day 1/Line 3

Spouse: Respondent number 001/Diary/Day 1/Line 4
Drank tea: Respondent number 001/Diary/Day 1/Line 4

However, although this categorization may be accurate, it is most likely that the first two categories would be grouped together as 'getting up'. 'Putting the kettle on' and 'making tea' might be coded as 'preparing a meal/drink', and the processes involved in cleaning out and lighting the fire might be grouped as 'fire chores' or classified with other household chores. Again, the family members could be described in terms of each relationship (husband, daughter, son, son-in-law, daughter-in-law, grandchild) or as broader categories such as partner, offspring, grandchild, in-laws, for instance.

On the other hand, it might be thought important to divide these categories in some way: for example, into positive and negative comments about family and neighbours or, as indicated in the marginal notes in Figure 10.2, 'visits from' and 'visits to' relatives. Also, the context in which the categories arise is likely to be important. The contextualization of categories involves noting down both the settings in which the categories arise and any other categories that are associated with a particular one. Clearly the level of categorization or coding is determined by the aims of the research – what *you* want to find out about. It might be that you decide to undertake a partial analysis rather than a full one; identifying categories that refer to your particular definition of health, for example. However, even this can be an extremely onerous and time consuming task, and many qualitative researchers have wished that they had carried out a survey when they reach this stage.

When all texts have been processed, the resulting lists are sorted, scrutinized and refined. This involves the inspection of the categories for completeness and redundancy. During this procedure, ideas and questions arise about the subject matter, and the texts might then be further scrutinized to test out any emerging patterns. These iterative aspects of qualitative analysis, mentioned at the beginning of this chapter, are continued until the researcher is satisfied that the data have been fully explored. However, as we will see below, interpretation also involves returning to the original texts and summaries to test explanations.

Although this and the previous stage are described as 'data analysis', many of the tasks undertaken are similar to the data processing procedures involved in quantitative research: the data are cleaned up and scrutinized, a coding scheme devised, and the data are coded ready for analysis. In the early stages of qualitative analysis, many of the procedures are concerned with the identification of variables and their possible values: coding. The difference, however, is that while undertaking these detailed textual processing procedures, the qualitative researcher is also using analytical skills to identify patterns and emerging themes in the data.

Data interpretation

As we have seen above, while processing and categorizing the texts, ideas about themes, patterns and relationships in the data gradually emerge. Data interpretation is specifically concerned with the identification and clarification of these features. This procedure involves not only the *description* of these, but may also go beyond this to attempt to understand and *explain* the patterns and relationships (generate theory).

The first stage in data interpretation involves the comparison of cases and categories, rather like the frequency distributions and cross tabulations carried out with quantitative data. Indeed, it is often possible to transform the categories to at least the nominal level of measurement. For example, if the text from all of the diaries reproduced by Townsend (1963) were to be analysed, we might look at the differences in lifestyle between older married couples and older single or widowed persons. And within this, we could look at differences between those with offspring living close by, or living further away, and those with no offspring. Alternatively, we might want to examine the subjective views about personal health status of those living in different housing conditions, with different income levels, or other aspects of life chances and history.

In order to make these comparisons, and to identify the patterns and relationships in the data, grids or matrices are often employed. These can take various forms. However, they are usually based on either of two formats: a category-by-category grid or a text-by-category grid. These are shown in Figure 10.3. In the first type of grid, category-by-category, the categories are listed in order across the top row of the grid (or spreadsheet) and down the first column. Categories that occur together in the text are checked off in their intersecting cell or box. In the example, text reference numbers have been used as the 'check' symbol. Here we see that in texts numbered 001, 030 and 012, categories 2 and 3 are mentioned together, and in text 0012, category 8 is also found in combination with categories 2 and 3. Tally methods other than text numbers can be used as appropriate. Once the grid is filled in, it will be possible to see how the categories interrelate, and the strength of this relationship: the more checks or 'hits' in a cell, the stronger or more frequent the relationship.

The second type of grid, text-by-category, is similar in layout to the previous one. However, here, the categories are only listed once, in either the first column or the first row depending on your preference. The other axis lists the text reference numbers. Thus 'number 008' has two mentions of category 2 and two of category 7. The 'number' can refer to a respondent (in interview or diary text, for instance), or an observation etc. As categories are checked off for each text, clusters or

A category-by-category grid

	Cat 1	Cat 2	Cat 3	Cat 4	Cat 5	Cat 6	Cat 7	Cat 8	Cat 9
Cat 1									
Cat 2									
Cat 3		001 030 012							
Cat 4					015 010				
Cat 5									
Cat 6									
Cat 7									
Cat 8		012	012						
Cat 9									

The shaded cells represent category intersection. Usually these would not be used. However, in certain instances, they might.

A text-by-category grid

	001	002	003	004	005	006	007	008	009
Cat 1									
Cat 2								✓✓	
Cat 3									
Cat 4									
Cat 5									
Cat 6									
Cat 7						✓✓✓		✓✓	
Cat 8						✓			
Cat 9									

Figure 10.3 *Examples of grids used in qualitative analysis*

patterns will emerge as the grid is filled in. This type of grid will help identify clusters of cases.

In an ongoing study of 'health alliances', the author and other colleagues used grids to examine the relationship between the organizational structures and the types of projects initiated by thirty UK Healthy Cities alliances (Payne and Sheaff, 1998). First, project categories were identified from an analysis of an open-ended question that asked for information about activities and projects undertaken in a particular time period. From this, sixty-two categories were originally identified. These were gradually refined to nineteen and, by using a category-by-category grid, it was possible to identify four activity clusters: community development; behavioural/lifestyle; strategic/structural; information provision. Finally, because it was mentioned so rarely – a significant finding in its own right – it was decided to drop 'information provision' in the further analysis.

A further category-by-category grid was then constructed. This listed the first three categories against organizational categories (lead agency; local authority type; year of establishment; WHO or non-WHO alliance; active involvement of local and health authority senior officers). The resultant grid showed a fairly clear pattern, so that overall strategies could be identified from the distribution of project types. These strategies were also related to particular organizational structures, and a typology could then be created.

The use of such grids and other devices might be seen as an oversimplification of the texts. In these, data reduction results in a large shift away from the reality or experiences that were the subject of the study. These devices, however, should be seen as merely heuristic devices: aids to the analytical process. The patterns and relationships that are identified by using such devices are checked and tested against the textual materials and the findings of existing studies. In addition, reference can be made back to respondents. These checks include looking for contradictory cases and evidence, and may be compared to the testing of a null hypothesis in quantitative analysis. However, here, the objective is not to demonstrate reliability by statistical significance, but to verify or modify by iteration until the researcher is sure that the findings are legitimate. This is often referred to as 'reaching *theoretical saturation*' (Sapsford and Abbott, 1992: 129).

An important part of this process is the analysis of the researcher's own reflexive accounts. As described earlier in this chapter, throughout the course of qualitative research, it is important to record the thoughts, ideas, actions and procedures that the researcher has or does. While this may help the researcher cope with the stresses of field work, the primary reason for doing this is so that these accounts can be subjected to analysis and scrutiny.

Visual analysis

Reversing the old adage, visual analysis is the process whereby a single image is translated into a thousand words! These data come in many forms, such as photographs, films, videos, paintings, drawings, cartoons and even graffiti – and photographs of graffiti. Such images have usually played a minor role in most social research, with its emphasis on word- and number-based data, despite the fact that, as people, we constantly look and see, as well as speak, write and listen. When visual images have been used, typically they have been in the form of one or two photographs that *illustrate* the physical environment, artefacts, or social activities of a 'society' (in anthropological texts) or a 'community' (in sociology). Sometimes films, and more recently video recordings, have been made to use in lectures about a particular topic or community. However, despite the fact that a considerable number of visual images have been made by social researchers, very few have been subjected to detailed analysis: exceptions include an analysis of family photographs by Chalfen (1998), Farran's (1990) analysis of pictures of Marilyn Monroe, and the study of tramps by Harper (1981).

One approach to visual analysis is through *semiological analysis*. *Semiotics* is based on the work of the Swiss linguist Saussure. Saussure saw language as a system of signs. A word was a *sign*. *Signs* are composed of two sub-constructs, the *signifier* and the *signified*. The *signifier* is the word as spoken by the speaker, and the *signified* is the word as understood by the listener. This approach can be applied to non-verbal communication systems as long as the object (the *signifier*) is seen. Thus a bunch of flowers can be a *signifier* for love, condolences, apologies, greetings, etc. The nature of the message (the *signified*) is determined by the cultural context in which it occurs. Hence, flowers do not signify anything naturally, only culturally. Those interested in semiotics should consult such texts as Barthes (1964) and Blonsky (1985).

This approach to visual analysis attempts to understand cultural signs and symbols by interpreting visual signifiers and any supporting text. Wetton and McWhirter (1998) give a report of this type of analysis in an evaluation of dental health education material for children aged four to seven. The material used various cartoon characters to convey the message of the importance of brushing teeth and the dangers of eating sugary products. One of the characters, 'Suzy Sugar', was depicted as a provocative, smiling, be-ribboned girl holding a lollipop with a bite taken out. Above this is written 'Suzy Sugar', and below her are the words 'Try to avoid her'. When the children were asked to interpret this cartoon, their understandings were very different from those intended by the (adult) creator. To the children, a smiling face signified 'good', and, given that she was eating a lollipop, some interpreted the message of the cartoon as 'eat lollipops'. The children were then told (verbally) that Suzy was trying to tempt them to be like her and eat sweets, but that this was bad. They were subsequently asked to draw their own versions of Suzy. All of these cartoons depicted an unsmiling girl with an 'ugly black mouth' (Wetton and McWhirter, 1998: 267).

It is important to recognize that visual awareness and research go much further than videoing a meeting or photographing bad housing. A whole range of visual materials can be quizzed for their meaning, again using the grid method. As an example of this, we can take the present author's visual analysis that described and interpreted the cultural signs in the work of a contemporary Scottish artist (Payne, 1991, 1994). First, images of the art works were each classified by noting down the following on a grid: the title (a textual signifier); the media used; the date produced; the size; the colours; the objects and symbols used (the visual signifiers); the researcher's initial feelings and interpretation (the signified). This study also involved analysis of face-to-face and telephone interviews with the artist, letters and other documents. The works were mostly highly complex, mixed-media structures (collages, constructions) that demanded a fairly detailed knowledge of contemporary and past life in the Scottish Highlands. By interpreting the many visual signifiers and the textual clues in the titles, the works were classified into three broad categories: the artist's childhood and family history; seafaring; and Highland history and literature. The following extract is from the results of this process. The picture,

Memories of a Northern Childhood, 1977, is his attempt to express some of this childhood experience. Like many of the works of this period, it is a mixed media box construction. Small in scale (48 × 35 × 15 cms), it represents the interior of a typical West Highland house with its tongue and groove wood panelling and dado rail. Inserted in a rack are small found and carved objects which recall his grandparents' home: a broken clay pipe, a cut throat razor, net holders and weavers. The viewer is drawn through the open shutters above the rack to a small slate relief of an old steam boat mounted in the familiar Maclean totem pole symbol: the upright fish net. The whole work conveys, partly through the richly stained wood, an air of warmth and happiness but also nostalgia and sadness: those days are gone forever. It is about growing up, an epitaph to childhood.

In contrast to the intimacy and warmth created by *Memories of a Northern Childhood*, *The Archaeology of Childhood*, produced twelve years later, is cold and more brutal. This work is about getting old. The pale blue-grey wash which covers the work and the thinness and fragility of the objects suggest cobwebs. It is like opening up a very old cupboard and finding everything covered in a pale grey coating of dust and spiders' webs. One can almost smell the mustiness. In this work the fish net and fish shovel totems have been brought inside and flank an inner cupboard. The cupboard contains carved toy soldiers which appear on the tops of the fish nets along with boat and fish symbols.

Both of these works are very personal reflections of childhood. Because of the symbols used and knowledge of the artist's background, they are easily recognised as being about a Highland childhood. However, the overall effect conveyed moves the works from the specific to the more general: this is how we all remember our childhood. (Payne, 1994: 99–100)

This form of analysis could also be applied to collections of old photographs, photographs that you might ask people in a community to take themselves, or children's drawings, for instance. You might first analyse them by noting down the objects and events depicted. These could then be interpreted using your own cultural knowledge, or you might ask the people who took or showed you the photographs what they meant to them. If this process was undertaken systematically for all the images collected, a detailed description and interpretation of the meanings could be developed.

Computer-assisted analysis

Throughout this chapter reference has been made to the use of computers in the transcription, indexing and analysis of qualitative data. Word processing and spreadsheet packages can be used for all or part of these procedures. For example, a word processing package could be used to search for particular words or phrases by using the 'find' facility. Each 'hit' could then be highlighted or separately recorded with reference details. These records could then be transferred to a spreadsheet to create indexes for each category identified. Alternatively, you could use the indexing facility that comes with the more sophisticated packages. Spreadsheet packages could also be used to construct grids and other matrices.

In addition to these fairly standard packages, a number of programs have been designed specifically as an aid to the analysis of qualitative data. The most widely known of these are *Ethnograph* and *NUD*IST*. These require a fairly high level of computer skill. They are also still at an early stage of development (when compared with the *SPSS* package, say), and are likely to be inappropriate for use by those who are new to qualitative research. While they can be used to carry out many of the more tedious parts of content analysis, coding and cross-referencing, for example, they are not a short cut, nor do they magically do the work for you. Indeed the danger here is that, by using them for this process, the researcher does not scrutinize the data in as much detail as in a manual search, and this has later implications for interpretation. On the other hand, they do accelerate analysis once data entry and coding have been done, and reduce the amount of subjective analysis needed in the interpretation of qualitative data. Those wanting to find out more about these packages should consult such texts as Fielding and Lee (1991), Gahan and Hannibal (1998), Grbich (1999), and Weitzman and Miles (1994).

Chapter summary

Qualitative data analysis is concerned with reducing largely unstandardized data to '*texts*' that can be coded into *concepts* and *categories*. Like other theoretical approaches to qualitative analysis, the *mainstream-traditional* approach is an extremely lengthy and demanding procedure involving data *transcription, inspection, coding* and *interpretation*. It is not an 'easy option' for those wishing to avoid statistics or wanting to have lots of 'cosy chats'. In addition to textual analysis, the chapter suggested ways in which *visual images* might be analysed and interpreted rather than being merely illustrative. This method is particularly suited to research involving young people.

Finally, the chapter considered the use of *computers* in qualitative analysis. Most people are likely to use word processing packages for text storage, and these (and spreadsheets) can also be an aid to analysis. However, they are not a short cut. Researchers must still undertake a detailed inspection of their texts to identify the categories and concepts that they will use in their interpretation.

Exercise

Carry out an analysis of the text from the diary entry in Townsend (1963) that is quoted in Chapter 6 (see p. 86). Those wishing to attempt further analysis could analyse all of the diary entries given in Annex 3 of the Townsend text.

PRESENTING THE EVIDENCE

The final stage of a research project is to 'tell the story' about it. You will be communicating to others not only the research findings but also the original aims and objectives, and the methods that you have used to collect the resulting evidence. Although sometimes one comes across research reports that are little more than ordered collections of all of the written outputs from particular projects (questionnaires, transcripts, tables etc.), this is not the recommended format. Such bundles are off-putting to all but the most dedicated reader, and they are likely to become merely temporary door jams gathering dust rather than contributions to knowledge.

Instead of this mass of paper, your report should aim to be a summary of the main issues uncovered by your research. This should be presented in such a way that your audience is able to understand clearly what you have discovered and the methods that you have used. Further, although the vast majority of reports are in a written form, they need not necessarily be so. Often visual displays, oral presentations, or a mixture of all three may be more appropriate.

This final chapter discusses how you might go about presenting your evidence in these different formats. This will be largely determined by the audience you wish to address and the nature of your findings. Your purpose for doing the research will also influence your presentation: does it have purely academic goals or is it intended to inform public debate, raise public awareness, or to have policy or practice implications?

Preliminary considerations

What do you want to say?

This question is concerned with the main message or series of messages that you wish to convey. When you have completed your analysis, you can write a list of your main findings. These should be grouped into broad areas relating to the topics that you listed at the beginning of your research. Sometimes, and always in exploratory research, topics will arise from the analysis itself. Within each topic area, your findings might be grouped into sub-categories. These should be ranked so that the most important points are made first, and in an order that moves logically from item to item. These topics can then be listed as a series of short words or phrases rather than long statements of findings. This framework can then form the basis of your presentation, because it covers everything about the research that you might wish to say, in a simple but structured and coherent way.

Table 11.1 shows one example of such a list of findings drawn up from the contents of *What You Said* (Healthy Sheffield, n.d.). Here we see that three broad areas are listed: What Affects Our Health; Health of People in Sheffield; Improving Our Health. Within each of these areas are a list of sub-topics or factors relating to the main heading. By creating such a list, you can begin to put a structure onto your mass of findings.

Table 11.1 *Example of a findings summary*

What Affects Our Health?
Income
Environment
Products and activities
Education
Social support
Social rights
Care
Workplace

Health of People in Sheffield
Women's health
Men's health
Children's health
Older adult's health
Health of black and minority ethnic communities
Health of people with disabilities
Lesbians and gay men
Young people's health

Improving Our Health
Community development
Organizational development
Education and training
Information and research
Planning for health
National and international advocacy

Source: Healthy Sheffield, n.d.

Who is it for?

The way in which you present your findings is determined, to a large extent, by your audience. The audiences that you might have to report to are likely to include one or more of the following: academic; professional group; employers; local or health authority; sponsors; community groups. A presentation to an academic audience is likely to be very different from that to a community group. Academics, for example, will probably be concerned with the contribution the work makes to the discipline. They will also be concerned with the validity, reliability or trustworthiness of the methods used, in addition to the findings. A community group, on the other hand, is more likely to be concerned with how the findings impact on the community, whether your findings confirm their own opinions, and the policy implications of the research.

Even the kinds of audiences we have identified can be broken down into more specific types, each of which may require a different presentation and could react in different ways. An academic group could be your seminar group, your tutors or examiners, a conference session, or an academic journal readership. Your presentations will be different in each case. If your presentation is to the local community, you need to decide whether this will be to the whole community or to individual community groups and organizations. At this stage it is worth making a list of the different groups that you want or need to inform, so that you can estimate how many different presentations you will have to make. This will give you a clearer indication of how much preparatory work will be involved.

In what form will you present it?

Your target audience and the nature of your findings will very much determine how you present your results. For example, if you have a considerable amount and variety of information to present, you should consider whether this would be best presented as a single presentation or as a series of 'topic' reports. Again, it might be that you want to keep people informed throughout your project by making interim presentations at different stages. Here, as a minimum, you will be expected to report to your supervisors and/or sponsors on a regular basis. In larger projects, seminar presentations will also be expected.

In determining the form of your presentation, you will have to decide on the best method of attracting and holding the attention of your audience(s). For instance, if you want to inform your local authority, community organizations and as wide a section of your community as possible, you might consider producing a number of different formats: a detailed presentation and a series of shorter topic or interim presentations. Avon Health's *Person-to-Person* project produced two report formats: a detailed report to each of four working groups who were involved in the project (Health Promotion; Primary Care; Acute Care; Accident and Emergency) and a summary report for participants (Shepherd, 1995). In the case of a university-funded research project on social deprivation that had been commissioned to have policy implications, the author wrote a formal report, an executive summary and a press release. These were accompanied by an oral presentation at a seminar held for local organizations and interviews with the press, television and radio. Finally, a paper was written for a conference, and academic journal articles were also published (Payne, 1995; Payne G. et al., 1996; Payne J. et al., 1996).

In these examples, the presentations took different forms for the different audiences. Exhibitions, photographic, slide and video presentations might also be appropriate for different groups. These could be used as a focus for a forum. Here, you would also need to prepare summary sheets or leaflets to hand out. When deciding on the format of your presentations, you should consider all of these different methods. In particular, it is worth looking at what others have done, and which of these have been successful and which have not.

Preparing a presentation

Whatever method you use to communicate your findings, there are a number of key points that need to be followed. The list of your findings grouped into topics should be used to guide your presentation. Using this, your aim should be to present a *clear, well argued and accurate* account of your findings in a *logically structured* way, using a *style appropriate* to your audience. Further, whatever your audience, you should try to avoid using jargon, and, if you do have to use technical terms, these should be clearly defined.

Writing a report

Writing a report is the most formal and structured method of presenting your project. A report usually takes a standard format. This would include:

- Introduction
- Methodology
- Findings
- Discussion
- Conclusions and Recommendations

Academic reports also usually include an *Abstract* of about 200–500 words at the beginning that summarizes the main findings and describes how they relate to existing knowledge. In reports to sponsors, local and health authorities, and other large organizations, the *Abstract* is replaced by an *Executive Summary*. This is usually no more than two or three pages in length, again at the front of the report. Here, you would list your main findings and recommendations, preferably as bullet points. The purpose of the abstract and the executive summary are basically the same: to let busy potential readers see your basic message, so that they can decide if they need to go further and read the whole document.

The *Introduction* is where the background to the research and the aims and objectives are discussed. In an academic report, this section should also include a *literature review*, reporting relevant findings and key ideas from earlier studies as a background to your work. This would be extensive in dissertations or monographs, forming a substantial part of the report, whereas in papers prepared for academic journals it might only cover the main contributions. In articles prepared for more popular journals the literature review is likely to be minimal.

The *Methodology* section, again, varies in length depending upon the type of report. This would be most extensive in dissertations, academic papers and monographs. Reports for sponsors and other public bodies should include sufficient information to allow readers to assess the appropriateness and, where necessary, the validity and reliability of the methods. It is sometimes not in the body of the report, but in an appendix at the end. As with the literature review, this section is either minimal or excluded in more 'popular' reports.

The *Findings* and *Discussion* sections are sometimes combined. If you decide to separate them, your findings should be described in a fairly straightforward manner. This section would include tables, graphs and other statistical outputs, where relevant. Your interpretation of these would then be discussed separately. You may prefer to present your findings and their interpretation together, and this can often be more meaningful. However, this is very much a matter of individual style.

In writing about each topic, you should try to avoid providing too many detailed tables and statistics. If necessary, these can be included in an *Appendix* or *Annex*. Topics can be illustrated by graphs, charts, photographs or drawings to make the text more easy to understand. An essential part of qualitative research reports is the inclusion of quotations from your observations, research diary and interviews. Here, it is important that the people from whom the quotations and descriptions have been taken are not identifiable. Usually interviewees are given fictional names, and identifying characteristics, such as age, number of children, etc. are changed. Two good examples of written presentations that use appropriate graphics and quotations to illustrate their findings are Bowling (1993) and Healthy Sheffield (n.d.). The reports were produced for different audiences, but both appeal to readers by their clever use of drawings and quotations.

The *Conclusions and Recommendations* to a report are where the findings are drawn together. Here, a summary of the main issues arising from the research are given, along with any policy or practice recommendations. After this section, formal reports include a *Bibliography*. This is now most often presented in the form used in this book (called the Harvard citation system). Here, all works cited in the report are listed alphabetically by author in the following form:

Dootson, S. (1995) 'An in-depth study of triangulation', *Journal of Advanced Nursing*, 22: 183–7.
Douglas, J. (1974) *Investigative Social Research: Individual and Team Research*. Beverly Hills, CA: Sage.
Dupuy, J. and Dupuy, P. (1980) 'Myths of the information society' in K. Woodward (ed.), *The Myths of Information Technology and Post Industrial Culture*. London: Routledge and Kegan Paul.

If your research has been carried out by more than one person, you will need to decide who is going to prepare the report. Is just one person going to take responsibility or will different people write different topics? Ideally, one person should take overall responsibility (as *'editor'*) even when a number of you may be contributing. This will ensure that the final version is written in the same style and that everyone produces their 'bit' on time. Once tasks are allocated, you should start writing the *first draft*. Usually, the main body of the report is written up first, and the Introduction and Conclusion are written last. At this stage, you will also need to produce a title page and a table of contents.

When you have completed the first draft, it is worth setting this aside for a short while before reading through it so that you can read it objectively. When you do read the draft, it is likely that you will want to make changes to both the content and the grammar and spelling. Although most word processing packages have spell-checks, it is important to read through the document yourself because there are many errors that cannot be detected automatically: for example, the spell-check will regard 'ant' and 'and' as both correctly spelt, but of course they mean different things.

Many academic reports go through five or more drafts before the author is satisfied. It is helpful, if possible, to circulate it to colleagues and friends for their critical comments. When all necessary changes have been made and any new ideas incorporated, you will have a final version for printing out, sending to a publisher or submitting to a journal.

Printing a report

Once you have decided on the text of your report, you will need to decide on its layout and how you are going to print it. This, of course, will be determined by your audience and your budget. However, whatever these are, it is usual for a report to be in typescript, and you will need at least two copies: one for yourself and one for your audience. Normally you will need more than this. Four copies are usually required for academic dissertations and journal papers, and publishers need at least two copies. The number of copies that sponsors, employers and other organizations require varies. You should find this out early on so that you have a clear idea of the total number of copies that you will need to print.

Whatever the audience, you should aim for a simple and clear layout. Academic reports, journal articles and published work are expected to be in a particular style. You will normally be informed of this but you should check if you are unclear. Reports for other agencies can have more varied layouts. Here, the many 'styles' that come with word processing and desktop publishing packages can be useful guides. However, do not be over ambitious or use too many different elements. If you keep to a maximum of two fonts – one for headings and one for text – using the bold and italic versions sparingly, your document will look more professional and be more readable than one that uses many different fonts and styles. For instance this:

Mary and her lamb
Mary had a little lamb, its fleece was white as snow. And *everywhere* that Mary went, the lamb was sure to go.

or this:

Mary and her lamb
Mary had a little lamb, its fleece was white as snow. And *everywhere* that Mary went, the lamb was sure to go.

Is more readable than this:

Mary
and

her lamb
Mary had a little **lamb**, its fleece was *white* as snow. **And** *everywhere* that
Mary went, the lamb was *sure* to go.

If you want to use graphic elements – photographs, drawings, clip
art, for example – you should use them sparingly. Here again it is best
to use only one or two different styles: photographs and line drawings,
or line drawings and coloured-in images, rather than all three. Some
reports that have been recently produced by community organizations
have tended to over-use these elements. The overall effect is too 'busy'
and looks amateur. If you do want an eye-catching layout that uses a
variety of elements, it is advisable to consult a qualified graphic
designer.

After deciding on your layout, you will need to reproduce it. This
will involve either photocopying or using an in-house or outside printing firm. As a general rule, if you need more than twenty copies of the
report, this should be done by a print firm. However, this is not a hard
and fast rule since the length of the report is also a factor. Binding also
has to be taken into consideration here, since some bindings ('perfect',
for instance) can only be done by a print house and are more expensive.
If you do decide to use an outside print firm, you should get a number
of quotes since charges can vary enormously.

Preparing a leaflet

The formal report discussed above is not really appropriate for a
general audience. Instead, community projects and Healthy Cities
initiatives have produced leaflets and fliers to keep members of the
community informed of their work. The content of these vary from
those giving an overview of the research to those that address a single
issue (for example, food; environment; young mothers; accidents).

The format of the leaflet determines how much information can be
conveyed, and you will have to decide on a layout before finalizing your
text. The most widely used format at the moment is the 'A4 bi-fold': a
sheet of A4 size paper folded into thirds (which takes two folds). This
gives up to six faces if printed on both sides. However, it is not usual to
use up all of the space with close-typed text. One face will be like the
cover of a report with a title. On the other five faces, the objective is to
convey your message using single words and short phrases and sen-
tences that can be quickly read and understood. As with questionnaires,
the language used should be simple and non-technical. Bullet points are
often used with different font styles (regular, bold, italic) and graphics
so that the reader's attention is drawn to the main points.

When drafting the text for these documents, you will have to decide on the main message that you wish to convey. This should then be reduced to about three or four topics per page, although some leaflets contain more. Try out a few different ways of writing the text because, as with reports, it is unlikely that you will get it right first time. Again, it is worth showing these to family, friends and colleagues for their comments.

Once you have decided on the wording, it is advisable to get these printed professionally. Although it is possible to print them yourself, professional printers are likely to be able to produce far higher quality documents than you can achieve with a home computer, printer and photocopier. Many printers have graphic designers who can advise on layout and images. Alternatively, they will have a range of layout styles that you can choose from. Charges for printing leaflets are very reasonable but it is worth getting quotes from two or three firms.

Verbal and visual presentations

You may decide that instead of, or in addition to, a formal written report, you would like to present your research findings at a meeting or seminar. Alternatively, you could consider putting on an exhibition of text and visual images. The type and style of the presentation is largely determined by your audience. An oral presentation to tutors, sponsors or statutory authorities, for instance, would be very different from that given to a group of school pupils or a community group because they will be interested in different aspects of your work. However, in all cases the aim should be to provide a clear and simple account that avoids jargon. In all cases you will need to write a script that summarizes your main findings. Other factors that need to be considered are whether to have a chairperson, and whether the presentation will be made by one person or a team.

Oral presentations should normally be limited to about an hour in length, which includes time for questions and answers. An oral presentation is a talk, not a reading from your report. You must prepare (with notes or charts to prompt your memory) a separate presentation, because a reading is boring and cold, and will 'turn-off' your audience. Be lively, stand up, and speak so that they can hear you and follow your argument. In the case of lengthy or complex reports, the presentation could consist of a number of talks covering different aspects, with breaks between each one. You should aim to cover a maximum of about five main points in each session. However interesting your research is to the audience, concentration does slip and details are lost. Varying the pace of presentation is important, as is the careful use of slides, overhead projections (OHPs) and other visual methods. Be careful, though, not to overdo the use of visual display material. They should be relevant and illustrative of the oral presentation rather than an alternative to it.

When planning your presentation, you should also consider how you will take questions. Questions are usually taken at the end but can also be taken during the presentation itself. When taken during the session, they do disrupt the flow and can lead to deviation from the script. This might not cause problems if you have decided on a flexible, open-ended approach. However, if you want to ensure that you can keep to your script, it is best to take questions at the end. Your audience should be informed of how questions will be taken before you begin. Here, having a chairperson helps. The role of the chair is to make sure that the presentation goes to plan and that questions are asked in an orderly way, so that you can concentrate on presenting your report.

If you decide to hold an exhibition, you will need to prepare a visual script or *storyboard*. A *storyboard* acts as a template for your display. First, you will need to decide what messages you want to convey and in what order you will convey them, although in an exhibition you cannot be sure that people will follow your order. You can then rough-out the type of image or text that is appropriate for each of these messages. When completed, the *storyboard* will look something like a strip cartoon. After you have selected the images and composed any accompanying text, you use the *storyboard* to guide the hanging of the display. Here again, you should aim for simplicity and clarity, although the use of collage, graffiti and other artistic techniques can be effective if used appropriately and professionally.

Publicity

A final task that needs to be carried out is concerned with the delivery and publicity of your work. You will have to decide how to inform your prospective audience that you have produced a document, or that there will be a meeting or exhibition about your research. How you go about this will be determined by the nature of your report and the type of audience you have in mind. If there is a need for any publicity about an academic monograph, this will be handled by the publisher. For local reports and meetings, publicity is up to you and any sponsors.

Sponsors or employers may only require that a specific number of copies are delivered to them by a certain time. Alternatively, they might send you a list of people who should receive a report of your work. In such instances your task is simply to deliver the report, preferably with a brief covering letter explaining the work and why they are being given a copy. For unsponsored work you would first need to draw up a list of individuals and organizations to whom you would like to send copies. You would then send copies of the report and a covering letter to those on your list. Similarly, leaflets could be delivered by post, by hand or bundles could be left at local outlets.

On the other hand, if you intend to promote the message of your research, to sell your report, or to hold a meeting or exhibition, you will need to advertise this. The form that this takes is again determined by your audience. For a general audience this might be through posters, advertisements in the local press or by word of mouth. The information that you need to include here is *what* it is about, *where* it will be held, and *when* it will be held (or, in the case of sales, what the report is about, from where they can obtain a copy, when it will be available, and the cost). These announcements should be simple and eye-catching. For specialist audiences you would first of all need to draw up a list of names before sending out the relevant information. Remember that in large organizations the front-line workers will not necessarily see a single copy sent to 'the Chief Executive', whereas small agencies may be able only to afford to buy one copy.

If you want your report to have a big impact, or you feel that it is newsworthy, then you will need to inform the media. This will entail writing a *press release* and being prepared to be interviewed. The format of a press release is fairly standard, not least because it helps the hard-pressed (local) journalist to use it! It should be boldly headed 'Press Release', followed by your research/group's name as a 'banner head-line' at the top of the first page. If you want it to be held back until a particular date (the date of your presentation or publication, for instance), you should state in bold 'Not to be released until (*date*)' or 'Embargoed until (*date*)'. You should use no more than two sides of A4 – double spaced – to make your pitch. Start with a headline: 'New Report Slams Traffic Pollution', or 'If You're Poor in Thistown, You Die 5 Years Early', or 'Gaps in Health Care Widen'. Be bold, to catch attention, but not sensational.

Take a lot of care in writing your first sentence, which ideally should 'tell the story in one go'. Use short paragraphs and simple language. Write it as a mini news story: busy journalists often include large chunks from press releases in their reports. Include some brief, repeatable quotations from the researcher or sponsor, so that journalists can give the impression that they did an interview: 'sound bites' are very powerful ways of communicating basic points.

You should also 'look for the hook'. Why should the media cover your story? What makes it newsworthy? Is it new, timely, a challenge to conventional wisdom, of interest to the media's own special audience? The present author's (1995) study of deprivation in Cornwall and Devon found that one ward in Plymouth – St Peter – had the worst deprivation score of any ward in England and Wales. That became 'the hook' to use in the press release, grabbing the media's attention. It played a key role in publicity, in the executive summary, and in a series of agency reports and funding bids that followed. St Peter was only a tiny part of the project and of the two counties, but it became the 'hook' on which communicating the rest of the research hung.

You can only cover a fraction of your hard work in a press release. If it is successful, journalists will follow it up, which gives you a second opportunity. You must therefore end the press release with the name of the person to be contacted, and a contact phone number. Although the media have their own agendas (and you do need to be careful of negative coverage), you should think in terms of making alliances that will result in at least some of your findings reaching a wider public.

The way to handle the media is sharply outlined by Polly Toynbee, the *Guardian*'s social affairs columnist, in the following extract from an interview for the British Sociological Association's newsletter, *Network*. Asked why researchers fail to get their message across, she replied

partly because they don't want to, and . . . [many of] those who are doing important and interesting work (a) write it very badly, (b) partly because of the funding system they are not funded to disseminate, so they don't and they haven't a clue how to anyway.

. . . They have no idea how newspapers work, no idea how to get a story out, they haven't the faintest idea how to write a summary on one side of a piece of paper so that a news editor might look at it. Or even someone like me who is rather more interested (and who might say 'gosh this is interesting'. Instead, a wodgey report arrives this fat [*gestures a very thick tome*] impenetrably written, with a bad summary – if one at all. It has no embargo date on it so you have no idea if someone else has written about it somewhere else, or not. A report should always be sent out at least two weeks beforehand with a firm embargo date on it. You need a press release stuck on the front, and a really good summary and a really good conclusion. If possible you have a Rowntree's boiled down 'Findings' (which are brilliant). Then researchers should ring journalists up who might be interested in that subject and remind them. These things are quite basic. . . . If there is important information and interesting stuff then it needs to get to policy makers, to government, to civil servants, and to journalists. I get a pile of mail this high . . . occasionally something comes up and I think 'yes – terrific!' and I write in my diary that this is coming out on such and such a day and take it home and I do read it. The health correspondent, the social services correspondent, also have their great piles and it's easier for them to get more news pieces into the paper than I can cover in my column. Usually once it does get into the newspaper, other people who are researching in the field, or policy makers, or other interested parties write in and ask for more information. We do act as important disseminators. It should be part of education for academics: What is your research for? Who is going to read it? . . . What use is it going to be? Who is going to make use of it? (Murphy, 1999: 22–3)

Implications for policy and practice

Unlike much academic 'pure' research, the production and dissemination of evidence is usually not the final stage in research concerned with the health needs of communities. Here there is an expectation that the findings will inform policy making or practice, since 'needs assessments are of no benefit in and of themselves' (Percy-Smith, 1996: 145). In this final section we will consider how this evidence has been used.

Throughout the 1990s, health ministers and statements in a number of Department of Health documents have stressed the importance of research findings to the policy making process. For example, in 1993 Mawhinney, then Minister for Health, maintained that

> decisions must be based on sound evidence about health needs . . . there is no substitute for detailed local investigations and these should underpin all major purchasing decisions (Mawhinney, 1993: 18)

However, this evidence is not likely to directly inform the policy making process.

> Translating research findings . . . into policy implications . . . is not a task for researchers alone . . . It is rather more likely to be successful if it is a collaborative exercise of stakeholders including researchers, policy makers, service managers and professionals, and financial experts . . . *Making research available and accessible does not ensure that it is used.* The research community and research funders can only play their part in what has to be a partnership in ensuring policy and services are soundly based. The major responsibility for utilizing research knowledge lies with the service community. (Department of Health, 1997b: 6–7; emphasis added)

That research findings are not necessarily used is well illustrated by the 1980 Thatcher government's treatment of the *Black Report*, and by successive Conservative governments' reactions to subsequent reports of inequalities in health (see, for instance, Barclay, 1995; Hill, 1995; Townsend et al., 1992). The Labour government which came to power in May 1997 reversed this attitude to health inequalities. In July 1997 an independent inquiry into inequalities in health was set up to review the latest evidence, and reported back in December 1998 (Department of Health, 1998b). Further, a needs-based approach was emphasized when Health Action Zones and Health Improvement Programmes were announced in the White Paper *The New NHS: Modern • Dependable* (Department of Health, 1997a).

These contrasting strategies clearly demonstrate the political context in which policy related research operates. Thus, the Department of Health's latest policy research strategy states that:

> There are many pressures for policy refinement and change – political direc-
> tion, legislative imperatives, and financial constraints – and in this sense
> research operates in a political context. (Department of Health, 1997b: 7)

It is still perhaps too early to assess what attitude the Blair government
will take towards research that does not support its political agenda –
'uncomfortable evidence', as Hunter (1994) calls it. But obviously only
the extremely naïve would expect that it would be treated impartially.

At the more local level, however, there are instances where research
has had a direct impact on policy and practice. Hunt (1993) shows how
research that established a link between damp mould and respiratory
problems impacted on housing policy in Glasgow, despite the 'dis-
pleasure' of the Scottish Office. Here, of course, there was a Labour-
controlled local authority and a Conservative central government. On
the other hand, without any obvious bias, the Health Education Authority based its 'Draw and Write Technique' for health promotion in
primary schools on research undertaken by Wetton and her colleagues
(Wetton and McWhirter, 1998). In contrast, the same organization was
less welcoming of an evaluation of community development techniques (Smithies and Adams, 1993). Many other successes and failures
at the local level can be found in Laughlin and Black (1995).

Conclusions

The importance of policy related research is illustrated by the body of
research that has had an impact on resource allocation, practice and
policy. Policy does not automatically result from research, but this is
more likely if evidence is based on appropriate and sound research
techniques and procedures. Further, the most likely way to 'make your
research matter' is to present it in as clear and understandable a way as
possible, ensuring that it gets to those patrons and key people who **can**
do something about it.

Exercise

Prepare a press release for any one of the case studies described in
this book.

CASE STUDIES

Reference has been made to many case studies in the main part of this book. Those that are particularly good examples of the research techniques described are summarized here. The descriptions are varied because of differences in the amount of methodological detail given in the studies. Costs have been given where known.

Involving the public in priority setting

(Bowling, 1993)
This study in the City and Hackney Health Authority area was funded by the King Edward's Hospital Fund for London. It was carried out by a team of social researchers based at St Bartholomew's Hospital Medical College.

Costs: £25,000 over 12 months, excluding interviewing and the principal researcher's and secretarial time. The community group survey cost £13,000; the postal survey, £2,000; the interview survey, £4,000 plus £3,000 (printing, postage, coding, data processing); the doctors' survey, £3,000.

Aims and objectives: to analyse the public's priorities for health provision; to compare priorities of different groups and those of the medical profession.

Methods: used a *mixed-method* approach – existing information (Census and other studies); self-completion questionnaire to community groups and group discussions; postal and interview survey of a random sample of district residents; postal questionnaire to members of the medical profession in the district.

Sample: 370 people in 27 groups; random sample of 454 residents taken from GP lists (with three reminders); 325 medical professionals (with three reminders).

Response: residents survey – poor response to postal questionnaire (10 per cent), increased to 77 per cent with interviews; medical professionals, 67 per cent.

Public involvement in purchasing priorities

(Richardson and Bowie, 1995)
This was a consultative process to find out the public's views on purchasing priorities. Used independent consultants to undertake the project.

Start up costs: £35,000–£40,000 per year.
Method: focus groups were consulted three times a year with 12 people in each group. Membership was on a staggered replacement basis, with 4 new members at each meeting. Meetings were held in the evenings with transport provided if needed. Members were paid £10 per session to cover expenses.
Sample: members recruited from local residents using a *quota sample* – stratified by gender, age and 'social background'.

Health needs of black and ethnic minority women

(Avan, 1995)
The project aimed to identify health issues affecting black and ethnic minority women and to raise awareness of these issues.

Method: existing statistical information; semi-structured questionnaire as a basis for *group discussions* with women from minority ethnic groups; one-to-one interviews with a wide range of those working with minority ethnic groups.
Sample: selected to ensure a range of backgrounds and experience.

Healthy Thamesdown

(Hall and Hannon, 1994)
This study used a *participative approach* and a broad definition of health. The area selected showed high levels of deprivation and ill health.

Steering group: 8 officers – 4 from Swindon Health Authority and 4 from Community Development, Thamesdown Borough Council.
Aims and objectives: to help service providers and purchasers meet the health needs of the local community and enabling them to participate in the decision-making process.

Method: existing census and health data; informal observations; individual interviews and group discussions were carried out by the locality team (120 people consulted).
Priority Search: 5 local people were trained as interviewers.

Winnall Neighbourhood Forum's community survey

(Winnall Neighbourhood Forum, 1993)
The project was part of a local community participation project initiated by Winchester Health Authority and funded by North and Mid Hampshire Health Commission and Winchester City Council. The project was facilitated by Winchester Health For All. The *community survey* was part of this project.

Planning group: local residents and organization representatives with survey experience.
Aim: to go beyond consultation by 'empowering people to identify and articulate their own needs'.
Methods: existing information; one-to-one interviews.
Topics: covered a wide range of *socio-economic* and *environmental* issues.
Interviewer: volunteers – 4 residents and 2 voluntary workers. Training was given by a local voluntary organization.
Sample: systematic random sample of 274 household (21 per cent).
Field work: took one month (afternoons, early evenings and weekends). Households were informed one week beforehand. Two call-backs.
Response rate: 40 per cent

Home helps

(Warren, 1990)
This is a *qualitative* investigation of the experiences of home helps caring for elderly people in Salford. The findings show how domestic, social care and nursing tasks are intermixed in predominantly low-skilled, part-time female employment. The 'social care' aspects, in particular, created feelings of attachment to and responsibility for those for whom they cared.

Method: *observations* and *group interviews* with 54 home helps over a 16 month period.

Information provision during confinement

(Kirkham, 1992)
This study investigated the ways in which information is requested by patients and given by staff in maternity delivery units.

Method: *observations* during labour and post-natal interviews with 90 patients; ante-natal interviews with 85 patients; observations of 5 domiciliary confinements and 18 GP Unit's patients.

Draw and write

(Wetton and McWhirter, 1998)
Wetton and McWhirter describe a number of studies that examined primary school pupils' perceptions of health education curricula. The studies used the *draw and write* technique instead of questionnaires to identify the development of children's understandings of health and health related behaviour. The Health Education Authority's 'Health for Life' programme was based on the findings of the largest study. This approach has also been used in Hungary and the former Yugoslavia.

Aim: to investigate children's perceptions of 'health' for health education programmes.
Methods: in the main study children were asked to make annotated drawings of how they kept themselves healthy. The texts were analysed qualitatively, using the drawings for elucidation.
Sample: main study – 22,600 4–9-year-olds in England, Wales and Northern Ireland.

School evaluation using photography

(Schratz and Steiner-Löffler, 1998)
This Austrian study attempted to discover primary school pupils' *evaluation* of their school's physical environment. The findings showed that pupils' feelings about physical areas of the school were very much influenced by their feelings about people and experiences that were associated with these areas.

Method: pupils were formed into teams of 4 or 5; each team was asked first to discuss and then *photograph* areas that they thought were good and bad; the teams used the resulting photographs to make annotated collages of their views.

The Devonport Initiative

(Lapthorne, 1996)
This was set up in 1992 to involve local people in health initiatives using a community development approach.

Costs: £150,000 per annum.
Method: *Rapid Appraisal* – existing information (problems with area definitions), interviews with 'key informants', and informal focus groups.

Dumbiedykes

(Murray and Graham, 1995)
This study used four methods of assessing the health needs of a GP practice's patients. The results showed variations in measurements of socio-economic factors and health status between the four methods. The researchers recommended the use of all four methods in a thorough needs assessment.

Method: existing information (Census and health authority small area statistics); practice held information; *Rapid Appraisal*; postal questionnaire (including the Nottingham Health Profile).
Response rate: 62 per cent to postal questionnaire.

Person-to-person

(Shepherd, 1995)
This study originated as a response to *Local Voices* and was influenced by methods of consulting the public used in Vermont, USA.

Costs: £10,000 per year, excluding staffing.
Method: a discussion document was circulated and followed up by 25 *focus groups* of people from voluntary and community organizations. These were facilitated by a range of people from the health authority and local groups.
Feedback: formal reports to the health authority working groups and 'user-friendly' summaries to those taking part.

Calderdale and Kirklees

(McHarg, 1996; Steering Group (Dewsbury), 1994, and 1995)
The health authority has adopted a strategic approach to public consultation that attempts to support an on-going dialogue with the public.

Running costs: £12,000 per year excluding staffing.
Method: 'talk back' *panels* (three questionnaires per year) and focus groups; ethnic group panels; *health forums*; community and planning groups.
Sample: the 'talk back' sample is drawn from the electoral register to ensure that it is representative of age, gender, ethnic and occupational groupings.

Healthy Sheffield

(Halliday, 1991; Healthy Sheffield, n.d.)
These are the outputs from a public awareness raising and consultation exercise conducted by Healthy Sheffield in 1991.

Aims and objectives: to explore the feasibility of involving the public in health issues.
Method: used a range of methods to inform the public on health and priority setting.
Response rate: 1620 responses from individuals and community organizations.
Field team: 300 people were trained to obtain feedback via meetings, forums, group and individual discussions.
Results: production of an *easy to read and well illustrated account* of the responses received.

Housing and health

(Hunt, 1993)
This is an account of two studies arising from a community group's slide-tape show about dampness and mould in public housing. The paper describes the *wider issues involved in policy related research* and the role of *lay people* and the *media*.

Aim: to investigate the relationship between health and housing.

Method: the first study involved a 'double-blind' survey – one of health and one of housing conditions carried out in 300 Glasgow council dwellings. A further study was undertaken in Glasgow, Edinburgh and three cities in England.

GLOSSARY

Medical terms

Birth rate/General fertility rate   Number of live births to women per 1000 women aged 15–44

Infant mortality rates

Stillbirth rate   Number of stillbirths per 1000 **total** births

Perinatal mortality rate   Number of stillbirths plus deaths to infants under 7 days per 1000 **total** births

Post-neonatal mortality rate   Number of deaths to infants aged 28 days to 1 year per 1000 **live** births

Infant mortality rate   Number of deaths to infants under 1 year per 1000 **live** births

Low birthweight rates

< 1500 g – very low birthweight < 2500 g – low birthweight   Number of live and stillbirths below the relevant weight **per 100 total** births

Mortality rates (death rates)

Crude death rate   Number of deaths per 100,000 population

Standard mortality ratio (SMR)   The actual (or observed) number of age- and gender-specific deaths compared with what would be expected if the national rates were applied, using the formula:

Observed deaths/Expected deaths $\times$ 100

100 is the national rate. Rates over 100 are above the national rate. An SMR of, say, 164 means that an area had 64 per cent (164 – 100) more deaths than the national rate, and a rate of, say, 60 means that an area had 40 per cent (100 – 60) fewer deaths than the national rate
NB: Death rates are also calculated for specific causes.

Morbidity rates (illness/disease)

Standard registration ratio for selected cancers (SRR)   These are calculated in the same way as the SMRs above to allow for comparisons to be made with the English rate

Incidence rates   The number of new cases of a disease that developed during a specific **period** of time

Prevalence rate   The number of people who have a disease at a specific **point** of time

Socio-economic terms

Economically active   Those people in paid employment plus those who are actively seeking work

Economically inactive   Those not included in the above – retired, looking after house, permanently sick, students etc.

Unemployed   A number of different definitions are used, which often leads to confusion. They are based on either:
The number of people **registered** as unemployed and receiving unemployment benefit
or
The number of people **actively seeking** work

Social class   An occupational classification used in many social statistics and reports – a hierarchical ranking based on the perceived degree of skill and social status of each occupation. The current classification is to be changed in the 2001 Population Census

Research terms

Data   A **plural noun**. These are information or 'facts'. They can be *hard* (presented as numbers) or *soft* (the text or audio recording of interviews, photographs, videos, etc.)

Method   This refers to any technique for collecting and analysing data

Methodology   Strictly defined, this is a particular way of thinking or looking at a topic or problem – the total approach to the subject, including the theoretical perspective. It is also mistakenly used to refer to a technique or group of techniques – these are the *methods*

Sample   A small number of units that are selected from a larger number of units (the population). If the sample is selected *randomly*, you can predict how similar (or representative) your sample is of the population, and carry out a range of statistical tests on your sample data

Qualitative   This term refers to data or techniques used to collect data that cannot be easily measured or counted

Quantitative   This term refers to data or techniques to collect data that can be counted

Questionnaire   A standardized list of questions used in surveys

Schedule   A questionnaire or less structured question list used by interviewers

Commonly used abbreviations

CHC	Community Health Council
DoH	Department of Health
GP	General Practitioner
HA	Health Authority
IMR	Infant Mortality Rate
NHP	Nottingham Health Profile
NHS	National Health Service
NHSME/NHSE	NHS Management Executive/NHS Executive
RA	Rapid Appraisal
SMR	Standard Mortality Ratio
WHO	World Health Organization
SF-36	Short Form-36

BIBLIOGRAPHY

Abbott, P. and Payne, G. (1992) 'Hospital visiting on two wards' in P. Abbott and R. Sapsford (eds), *Research into Practice: a Reader for Nurses and the Caring Professions*. Buckingham: Open University Press.

Abbott, P., Bernie, J., Payne, G. and Sapsford, R. (1992) 'Health and material deprivation in Plymouth' in P. Abbott, and R. Sapsford (eds), *Research into Practice: a Reader for Nurses and the Caring Professions*. Buckingham: Open University Press.

Avan, G. (1995) *Perceived Health Needs of Black and Ethnic Minority Women: An Exploratory Study*. Glasgow: Community Support Unit, Healthy Glasgow.

Bales, R.F. (1950) *Interaction Process Analysis: a Method for the Study of Small Groups*. Reading, MA: Addison–Wesley.

Barclay, P. (1995) *Inquiry into Income and Wealth*, Vol. 1. York: Joseph Rowntree Foundation.

Barthes, R. (1964) *Elements of Semiology*. New York: The Noonday Press.

Bell, C. and Newby, H. (1971) *Community Studies*. London: George Allen and Unwin.

Bell, J. (1987) *Doing Your Research Project: a Guide for First-Time Researchers in Education and Social Science*. Milton Keynes: Open University Press.

Benzeval, M., Judge, K. and Whitehead, M. (eds) (1995) *Tackling Inequalities in Health*. London: King's Fund.

Blonsky, M. (ed.) (1985) *On Signs*. Oxford: Blackwell.

Bond, J. and Carstairs, V. (1982) *Services for the Elderly*. Edinburgh: The Scottish Home and Health Department.

Bottoroff, J. (1994) 'Using videotaped recordings in qualitative research' in J. Morse (ed.), *Critical Issues in Qualitative Research Methods*. Thousand Oaks, CA: Sage.

Bowling, A. (1993) *What People Say About Prioritising Health Services*. London: King's Fund Centre.

Bowling, A. (1995) *Measuring Disease*. Buckingham: Open University Press.

Bowling, A. (1997) *Measuring Health: A Review of Quality of Life Measurement Scales*. Buckingham: Open University Press.

Bowling, A., Leaver, J. and Hoekel, T. (1988) *The Needs and Circumstances of People Aged 85+ Living at Home in City and Hackney*. London: City and Hackney Health Authority.

Bradshaw, J. (1972) 'A taxonomy of social need' in G. Mclachlan (ed.), *Problems and Progress in Medical Care*. Oxford: Nuffield Provincial Hospital Trust.

Brazier, J.E., Harper, R., Jones, N., O'Cathain, A., Thomas, K., Usherwood, T. and Westlake, L. (1992) 'Validating the SF-36 health survey questionnaire: a new outcome measure for primary care', *British Medical Journal*, 305: 160–4.

Brooker, C. (1993) 'Unplanned interactions between nurses and patients' visitors: an observational study in a renal ward'. Dissertation, School of Advanced Nursing, North East Surrey College of Technology.

Burton, P. (1993) *Community Profiling: a Guide to Identifying Local Need*. Bristol: SAUS.

Caro, F. (1981) 'Demonstrating community-based long-term care in the United States: an evaluative research perspective' in E.M. Goldberg and N. Connelly (eds), *Evaluative Research and Social Care*. London: Heinemann for PSI.

Carstairs, V. and Morris, R. (1989) 'Deprivation: explaining differences in mortality between Scotland and England and Wales', *British Medical Journal*, 299: 886–9.

Chalfen, R. (1998) 'Interpreting family photographs as pictorial communication' in J. Prosser (ed.), *Image-based Research*. London: Falmer.

Cohen, P.A. (ed.) (1982) *Belonging: Identity and Social Organisation in British Rural Cultures*. Manchester: Manchester University Press.

Compass (1996) *The Compass Handbook*. Leeds: Policy Research Institute, Leeds Metropolitan University.

Curtice, L. (1993) 'The WHO Healthy Cities Project in Europe' in J. Davies and M. Kelly (eds), *Healthy Cities: Research and Practice*. London: Routledge.

Denman, J. and McDonald, P. (1996) 'Unemployment statistics from 1881 to the present day', *Labour Market Trends*, January: 5–15.

Denzin, N. (1970) *The Research Act: a Theoretical Introduction to Sociological Methods*. Englewood Cliffs, NJ: Prentice Hall.

Department of the Environment (1983) *Urban Deprivation*. Information Note 2, London: DoE.

Department of the Environment (1995) *1991 Deprivation Index: a Review of Approaches and a Matrix of Results*. London: HMSO.

Department of the Environment, Transport and the Regions (1998) *Index of Local Deprivation*. London: DETR.

Department of Health (1993) *Implementing Community Care: Population Needs Assessment Good Practice Guide*. London: Department of Health.

Department of Health (1997a) *The New NHS. Modern • Dependable*. London: The Stationery Office. Cm. 3807.

Department of Health (1997b) *Policy Research Programme*. London: Department of Health.

Department of Health (1997c) 'Baroness Jay says research and development is vital', *Press Release*: 97/411.

Department of Health (1998a) *Our Healthier Nation. A Contract for Health*. London: The Stationery Office. Cm. 3852.

Department of Health (1998b) *Independent Inquiry into Inequalities in Health* (Acheson Report). London: The Stationery Office.

Douglas, J.W.B. (1981) 'The contribution of long-term research to social medicine' in F. Schulsinger, S. Mednick and J. Knop (eds), *Longitudinal Research: Methods and Uses in Behavioural Science*. Hingham, MA: Martinus Nijhoff.

Doyal, L. and Gough, I. (1991) *A Theory of Human Need*. London: Macmillan.

Farren, D. (1990) 'Analysing a photograph of Marilyn Monroe' in L. Stanley (ed.), *Feminist Praxis: Research Theory and Epistemology in Feminist Sociology*. London: Routledge.

Fielding, N. and Lee, R. (1991) *Using Computers in Qualitative Research*. London: Sage.

Foreman, A. (1996) 'Health needs assessment' in J. Percy-Smith (ed.), *Needs Assessment in Public Policy*. Buckingham: Open University Press.

Gahan, C. and Hannibal, M. (1998) *Doing Qualitative Research Using QSR NUD*IST*. London: Sage.

Garrett, A., Ruta, D., Abdalla, M., Buckingham, K. and Russell, I. (1993) 'The SF36 health survey questionnaire: an outcome measure suitable for routine use within the NHS', *British Medical Journal*, 306: 1440–4.

Goldberg, E.M. and Connelly, N. (1981) *Evaluative Research and Social Care*. London: Heinemann for PSI.

Goldblatt, P. (ed.) (1990) *Longitudinal Study: Mortality and Social Organisation 1971–81*. OPCS Series LS Newsletter, 6. London: HMSO.

Gordon, D. and Forrest, R. (1995) *People and Places 2: Social and Economic Distinction in England*. Bristol: SAUS.

Gordon, V. (1992) 'Treatment of depressed women by nurses', in P. Abbott and R. Sapsford (eds), *Research into Practice*. Buckingham: Open University Press.

Grbich, C. (1999) *Qualitative Research in Health: an Introduction*. London: Sage.

Hall, W. and Hannon, G. (1994) *The Locality Project in Park and Walcot East*. Swindon: Healthy Thamesdown.

Halliday, M. (ed.) (1991) *Our City, Our Health*. Sheffield: Healthy Sheffield.

Harding, S. (1995) 'Social class differences in mortality of men, recent evidence from the OPCS Longitudinal Study', *Population Trends*, 80: 31–7.

Harper, D. (1981) *Good Company*. Chicago: University of Chicago Press.

Harrison, B. (1996) ' "Tells a Story": Uses of the Visual in Sociological Research', in E. S. Lyon and J. Busfield (eds), *Methodological Imaginations*. Basingstoke: Macmillan.

Hawtin, M., Hughes, G. and Percy-Smith, J. (1994) *Community Profiling: Auditing Social Need*. Buckingham: Open University Press.

Healthy Sheffield (not dated) *What you Said: a Summary of the Response to Our City – Our Health Consultation*. Sheffield: Healthy Sheffield.

Hill, J. (1995) *Inquiry into Income and Wealth*, Vol. 2. York: Joseph Rowntree Foundation.

Hunt, S. (1993) 'The relationship between research and policy: translating knowledge into action' in J. Davies and M. Kelly (eds), *Healthy Cities: Research and Practice*. London: Routledge.

Hunt, S., McEwen, J. and McKenna, S. (1986) *Measuring Health Status*. London: Croom Helm.

Hunter, D. (1994) 'Social research and health policy in the aftermath of the NHS reforms' in J. Popay and G. Williams (eds), *Researching the People's Health*. London: Routledge.

James, N. (1992) 'A postscript to nursing' in P. Abbott and R. Sapsford (eds), *Research into Practice: a Reader for Nurses and the Caring Professions*. Buckingham: Open University Press.

Jarman, B. (1983) 'The identification of underprivileged areas', *British Medical Journal*, 286: 1705–9.

Jenkinson, C. (1997) *Assessment and Evaluation of Health and Medical Care*. Buckingham: Open University Press.

Kirkham, M. (1992) 'Labouring in the dark' in P. Abbott and R. Sapsford (eds), *Research into Practice: a Reader for Nurses and the Caring Professions*. Buckingham: Open University Press.

Krueger, R.A. (1994) *Focus Groups: a Practical Guide for Applied Research*, 2nd edn. Thousand Oaks, CA: Sage.

Krueger, R.A. and King, J. (1998) *Involving Community Members in Focus Groups*. Thousand Oaks, CA: Sage (Focus Group kit, 5).

Lapthorne, D. (1996) 'Deprivation, community development and health' in P. Burton and L. Harrison (eds), *Identifying Local Health Needs*. Bristol: Policy Press.

Laughlin, S. and Black, D. (eds) (1995) *Poverty and Health: Tools for Change*. Birmingham: Public Health Alliance.

Maconachie. M. (1997) Personal communication.

Marmot, M. and Theorell, T. (1988) 'Social class and cardiovascular disease', *International Journal of Health Services*, 18(4): 659–74.

Marmot, M., Davey Smith, G., Stansfield, S., Patel, C., North, F., Head, J., White, I., Brunner, E. and Feeney, A. (1991) 'Health inequalities among British civil servants: the Whitehall II Study', *Lancet*, 337: 1387–93.

Marmot, M., Shipley, M. and Rose, G. (1984) 'Inequalities in death – specific explanations of a general pattern?', *Lancet*, 5 May: 1003–6.

Mawhinney, B. (1993) 'The vision for purchasing' in B. Mawhinney and D. Nichols, *Purchasing for Health: a Framework for Action*. Leeds: NHS Management Executive.

McGhee, J. and McEwen, J. (1993) 'Evaluating the Healthy Cities Project in Drumchapel, Glasgow', in J. Davies and M. Kelly (eds), *Healthy Cities: Research and Practice*. London: Routledge.

McHarg, K. (1996) 'A strategic approach to public consultation', paper presented to *Consulting the Public on Health Care*, 6–7 June. Bristol: School for Policy Studies.

McLoone, P. and Boddy, F. (1994) 'Deprivation and mortality in Scotland, 1981–1991', *British Medical Journal*, 309: 1465–70.

Merton, R.N., Fiske, M. and Kendall, P.L. (1956) *The Focused Interview*. Glencoe, II: Free Press.

Morgan, D.L. (1997) *Focus Groups in Qualitative Research*, 2nd. edn. London: Sage (Qualitative Research Methods, vol. 16).

Morgan, D.L. (1998) *The Focus Group Guide Book*. Thousand Oaks, CA: Sage (Focus Group Kit, 1).

Morgan, D.L. and Krueger, R.A. (1997–8) *The Focus Group Kit* (6 vols). Thousand Oaks, CA: Sage.

Morris, R. and Carstairs, V. (1991) 'Which deprivation? A comparison of selected deprivation indexes', *Journal of Public Health Medicine*, 13: 318–26.

Murphy, L. (1999) 'Interview: Polly Toynbee', *Network, Newsletter of the British Sociological Association*, 72, January: 20–3.

Murray, S. and Graham, C. (1995) 'Practice based health needs assessment: use of four methods in a small neighbourhood', *British Medical Journal*: 1443–8.

Neve, H. (1996) 'Community assessment in general practice' in P. Burton and L. Harrison (eds), *Identifying Local Health Needs*. Bristol: Policy Press.

NHS Executive (1998) *Information for Health*. Leeds: NHSE.

NHS Management Executive (1991) *Assessing Health Care Needs*. Discussion paper. London: NHSME.

NHS Management Executive (1992) *Local Voices: the Views of Local People in Purchasing for Health*. London: NHSME.

Ong, B. and Humphris, G. (1994) 'Prioritising needs with communities' in J. Popay and G. Williams (eds), *Researching the People's Health*. London: Routledge.

ONS/CLS (1998) *Longitudinal Studies Newsletter*. 19 December. London: The Stationery Office.

Oppenheim, A.N. (1992) *Questionnaire Design, Interviewing and Attitude Measurement*. London: Pinter.

Pawson, R. and Tilley, N. (1997) *Realistic Evaluation*. London: Sage.

Payne, G. (1996) 'Imagining the community: some reflections on the community study as a method' in E.S. Lyon and J. Busfield (eds), *Methodological Imaginations*. Basingstoke: Macmillan.

Payne, G. (1998) Personal communication.

Payne, G., Payne, J. and Hyde, M. (1996) 'Refuse of all classes'? Social indicators and social deprivation' in *Sociological Research Online*, 1, 1, 3, <http://www.socresonline.org.uk/socresonline/1/1/3.html>

Payne, J. (1978) 'Talking about children: an examination of accounts about reproduction and family life', *Journal of Biosocial Science*, 10(4): 367–74.

Payne, J. (1991) 'Individual constructs of cultural identity with special reference to the work of Will Maclean'. Dissertation, University of Plymouth, Exeter campus. Microfiche.

Payne, J. (1994) 'Will Maclean', *Edinburgh Review*, 91: 98–115.

Payne, J. (1995) *Interpreting the Index of Local Conditions: Relative Deprivation in Devon and Cornwall*. Plymouth: Plymouth Business School, University of Plymouth.

Payne, J. and Sheaff, M. (1998) *Strategies and Organisations: Tackling Inequalities in UK Healthy Cities*. Research Report. Plymouth: Department of Sociology, University of Plymouth: xerox.

Payne, J., Payne, G. and Hyde, M. (1996) 'Who doesn't get what? Deprivation and class' in W. Bottero (ed.), *Post Class Society, Proceedings of the Cambridge Stratification Seminar 1995*. Cambridge: Sociological Research Group.

Percy-Smith, J. (ed.) (1996) *Needs Assessment in Public Policy*. Buckingham: Open University Press.

Percy-Smith, J. and Sanderson, I. (1992) *Understanding Local Needs*. London: Institute for Public Policy Research.

Phillimore, P., Beattie, A. and Townsend, P. (1994) 'Widening inequalities of health in Northern England, 1981–1991', *British Medical Journal*, 308: 1125–8.

Plymouth and District Community Health Council (not dated) *Survey of Ambulance Use*. Plymouth: Plymouth CHC.

Pocock, S., Shaper, A., Cook, D., Packham, R., Lacey, R., Powell, P. and Russell, P. (1980) 'British Regional Heart Survey: geographical variations in cardiovascular mortality and the role of water quality', *British Medical Journal*, 280: 1243–9.

Priority Search (1992) *What Would Make Bootle a Better Place to Live in?* Report commissioned by Sefton Metropolitan Borough Council. Sheffield: Priority Search Unit, Sheffield City Council.

Priority Search (1994) *What Would Improve Your Health, Happiness and Well-being?* Swindon: Healthy Thamesdown.

Richardson, A. and Bowie, C. (1995) 'Public opinion', *Health Service Journal*, 11 May: 25–6.

Sainsbury, S. (1973) *Measuring Disability*. London: Bell.

Sapsford, R. and Abbott, P. (1992) *Research Methods for Nurses and the Caring Professions*. Buckingham: Open University Press.

Sarantakos, S. (1993) *Social Research*. Basingstoke: Macmillan.

Schratz, M. and Steiner-Löffler, U. (1998) 'Pupils using photographs in school-evaluation' in J. Prosser (ed.), *Image-based Research*. London: Falmer.

Shepherd, M. (1995) 'Self service', *Health Service Journal*, 27 April: 24–5.

Shepperd, S., Doll, H. and Jenkinson, C. (1997) 'Randomised Controlled Trials' in C. Jenkinson (ed.), *Assessment and Evaluation of Health and Medical Care*. Buckingham: Open University Press.

Silverman, D. (1993) *Interpreting Qualitative Data*. London: Sage.

Silverman, D. (1997) 'The logics of qualitative research' in G. Miller and R. Dingwall (eds), *Context and Method in Qualitative Research*. London: Sage.

Smithies, J. and Adams, L. (1993) 'Walking the tightrope: issues in evaluation and community participation for health for all' in J. Davies and M. Kelly (eds), *Healthy Cities: Research and Practice*. London: Routledge.

Steering Group for the Health Panel for Minority Ethnic Communities in and around Dewsbury (1994) *Internal Report*. Dewsbury: xerox.

Steering Group for the Health Panel for Minority Ethnic Communities in and around Dewsbury (1995) *Internal Report*. Dewsbury: xerox.

Townsend, P. (1962) *The Last Refuge: a Survey of Residential Institutions and Homes for the Aged in England and Wales*. London: Routledge.

Townsend, P. (1963) *The Family Life of Old People*. Harmondsworth: Penguin.

Townsend, P. (1979) *Poverty in the United Kingdom*. Harmondsworth: Penguin.

Townsend, P. and Davidson, N. (1982) *Inequalities in Health: the Black Report*. Harmondsworth: Penguin.

Townsend, P., Davidson, N. and Whitehead, M. (eds) (1992) *Inequalities in Health: the Black Report and the Health Divide*, Harmondsworth: Penguin.

Townsend, P., Phillimore, P. and Beattie, A. (1988) *Health and Deprivation: Inequalities in the North*. London: Croom Helm.

Tsouros, A. (ed.) (1990) *WHO Healthy Cities Project: a Project Becomes a Movement – Review Of Progress, 1987–1990*. Milan: SOGESS.

Wall, W.D. and Williams, H.C. (1970) *Longitudinal Studies and the Social Sciences*. London: Heinemann.

Warren, L. (1990) '"We're home helps because we care": The experience of home helps caring for elderly people' in P. Abbott and G. Payne (eds), *New Directions in the Sociology of Health*. Basingstoke: Falmer.

Weitzman, E. and Miles, M. (1994) *Computer Programs for Qualitative Data Analysis*. Thousand Oaks, CA: Sage.

Wetton, N. and McWhirter, J. (1998) 'Images and curriculum development in health education' in J. Prosser (ed.), *Image-based Research*. London: Falmer.

Whitehead, M. (1988) *The Health Divide*. Harmondsworth: Penguin.

Winnall Neighbourhood Forum (1993) *What about Winnall?* Interim Report. Winchester: Winnall Neighbourhood Forum.

Young, M. and Willmott, P. (1957) *Family and Kinship in East London*. London: Routledge and Kegan Paul.

Statistical Reports

The following UK statistical reports, produced annually or quarterly, might also be consulted.

Family Expenditure Survey
General Household Survey
Health and Personal Social Services Statistics
National Food Survey
Population Census Reports
Population Trends
Regional Trends
Social Trends
The New Earnings Survey

NAME INDEX

SUBJECT INDEX